Praise for
Pilates for Runners

"In *Pilates for Runners,* Sean Vigue shows you how to harness Pilates' most powerful benefits: greater strength and mobility, improved breathing and coordination, and more drive in every stride. Discover how Pilates can help you move with confidence, prevent common injuries and keep you running for years to come."

—Brooke Siler, author of *New York Times* bestseller *The Pilates Body*

"As endurance athletes, we often chase miles and intensity, but true performance comes from body awareness, control and efficient movement. *Pilates for Runners* gives runners the tools to move better, stay injury-free, and build the kind of durability that lasts beyond the finish line."

—Andrejs Birjukovs, ultra-endurance athlete, resilience coach and author of *The Resilient Athlete*

"Runners, like most athletes, tend to do too much of what they enjoy and not enough of what allows them to continue to be able to do what they enjoy. Filling their training gaps with practices like Pilates enables you them to do what they enjoy at a higher level with a lower risk of injury. There's no person I'd recommend more than Sean Vigue when it comes to Pilates."

—Dean Pohlman, founder of Man Flow Yoga and bestselling author of *Yoga Fitness for Men* and *Yoga for Athletes*

PILATES FOR RUNNERS

PILATES
FOR
RUNNERS

THE ULTIMATE GUIDE TO BUILDING STRENGTH,
MOBILITY & ENDURANCE FOR BETTER PERFORMANCE

SEAN VIGUE
FOREWORD BY
DEAN KARNAZES

Hatherleigh Press, Ltd.
62545 State Highway 10, Hobart, NY 13788, USA
hatherleighpress.com

PILATES FOR RUNNERS

Library of Congress Cataloging-in-Publication Data is available.
ISBN: 978-1-961293-50-2

Cover and interior design by Carolyn Kasper
Photography by Morrison Media, LLC

The authorized representative in the EU for product safety and compliance
is Catarina Astrom, Blästorpsvägen 14, 276 35 Borrby, Sweden.
info@hatherleighpress.com

Printed in the United States

10 9 8 7 6 5 4 3 2 1

To the memory of our beautiful dog, Addie.

She appeared in thousands of my videos

and is sorely missed every day.

We love you.

"Every moment of your life can be

the beginning of great things."

—Joseph Pilates

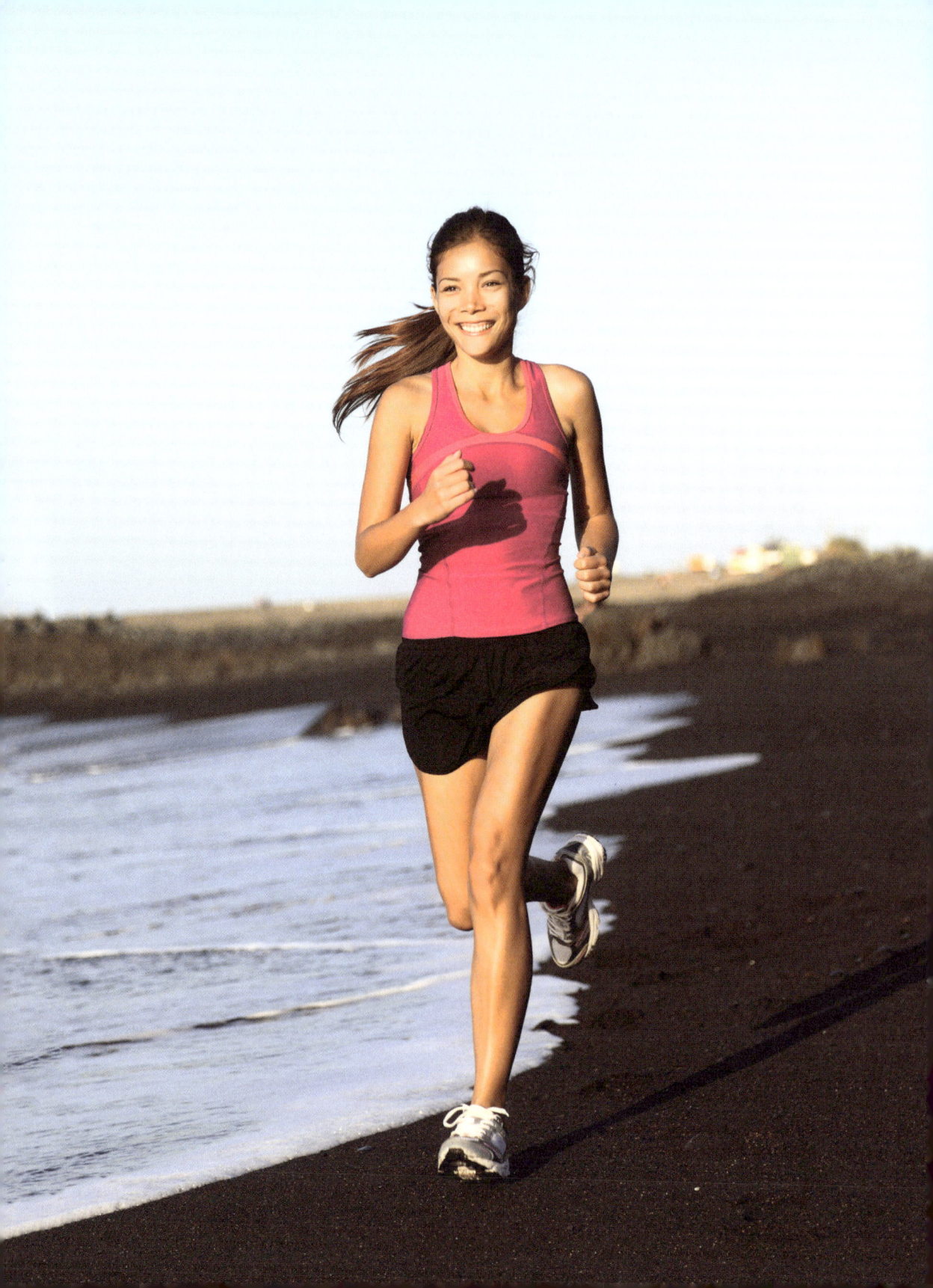

Contents

Foreword
by Dean Karnazes

I've long been an advocate of runners strengthening their overall body. To me, for a runner just to run is a recipe for injury and decreased running longevity. This, of course, begs the question: how to strengthen a runner's body?

Pilates is a proven exercise technique that has been shown to offer a myriad of benefits to a runner. These include greater strength, better endurance, improved flexibility, more efficient breathing, and an enhanced mind-body connection. And unlike weight training, Pilates has a lower risk of injury.

So why don't more runners embrace Pilates? Perhaps I can answer this question, from firsthand experience. I'll be honest—I was skeptical. To me, Pilates was something older people did because they didn't have the strength or stamina to do anything more. But I tried to keep an open mind on the subject and decided to try a Pilates session with my mom. The outcome?

I got my ass kicked! Not only was my flexibility atrocious, I also discovered certain muscle sets were significantly underdeveloped—despite years of weight room training.

I've now come to embrace Pilates as an essential training tool and exercise. And as I have, I've heard from other runners that have said Pilates helped them overcome some common running injuries like runner's knee, shin splints, Achilles tendinitis and IT band syndrome. Thankfully, I have never experienced any of these, and I believe Pilates has played a prophylactic role in avoiding these setbacks.

In *Pilates for Runners*, author Sean Vigue details everything a runner needs to know about creating an exercise regime and how to incorporate Pilates into a lifestyle, one in which movement and breathing helps build a stronger you. His instructions are clear, illustrative and—most of all—easy-to-follow. And if you look at him, it is clear that he practices what he preaches. The results don't lie.

So please, if you've been resistant to trying Pilates yourself, put down your defenses and take a leap of faith. Whether you run great distances, modest distances, or are just starting out, *Pilates for Runners* is an indispensable resource to keep you going, mile after mile.

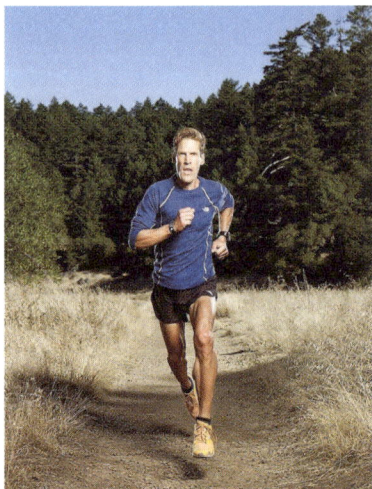

Named by *TIME Magazine* as one of the "100 Most Influential People in the World," Dean Karnazes has pushed his body and mind to inconceivable limits. Among his many accomplishments, he has run 50 marathons, in all 50 US states, in 50 consecutive days. He's run across Death Valley in the middle of summer, and he's run a marathon to the South Pole. An ESPN ESPY winner and 3-time recipient of Competitor magazine's Endurance Athlete of the Year award, Dean has served as a US Athlete Ambassador in overseas sports diplomacy envoys to Central Asia and South America. He's twice carried the Olympic Torch and is a recipient of the President's Council on Sports, Fitness and Nutrition Lifetime Achievement Award. A *New York Times* bestselling author, Dean has written several books including *Ultramarathon Man, 50/50, RUN!, The Road to Sparta,* and *A Runner's High*. He is a frequent speaker and panelist at many running and sporting events worldwide.

Introduction

Calling all runners! Ready to uncover a secret weapon to supercharge your stride, boost your breathing, slash your recovery time, and help you smoke your personal bests? Good—because what you're holding isn't just a book, it's your *new daily training partner*. And guess what? It's not fancy, it's not complicated—it's just you, your mat, and the powerhouse workout known as **Mat Pilates**.

These exercises are built to strengthen your core, improve posture, increase flexibility, and give you that smooth, injury-free stride that makes other runners jealous. You're reading this for a reason, and I bet your body's already saying, *"Let's go!"* Flip ahead and you'll find 40 game-changing exercises, 10 delicious stretches, and 15 workouts that are as fun as they are effective.

Words are great, but let's be honest—**the workouts are where the real magic happens.** You can read about the Pilates Hundred or Breaststroke all day long, but until you do them, they're just fancy names. It's the movement—the sweat, the control, the breathing, the challenge that transforms your body and takes your running, jogging, sprinting, trail running, or power walking to the next level. (Yes, we'll break those down in just a bit.)

You're a runner. That means you're a person of action, not fluff. I know you didn't pick up this book for a never-ending motivational speech—you're here to get faster, stronger, and smoother, and you want to do it now. I don't blame you.

Here's the truth: **Pilates and running are like peanut butter and jelly** (or jam; jam tastes better). You wouldn't expect them to go together, but when they do?

Total game-changer.

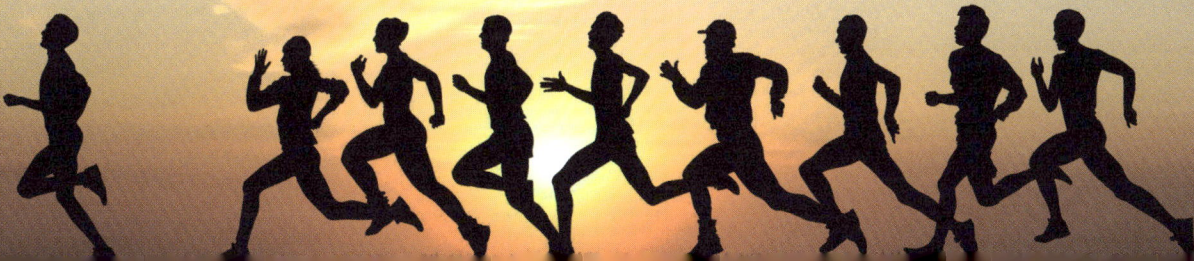

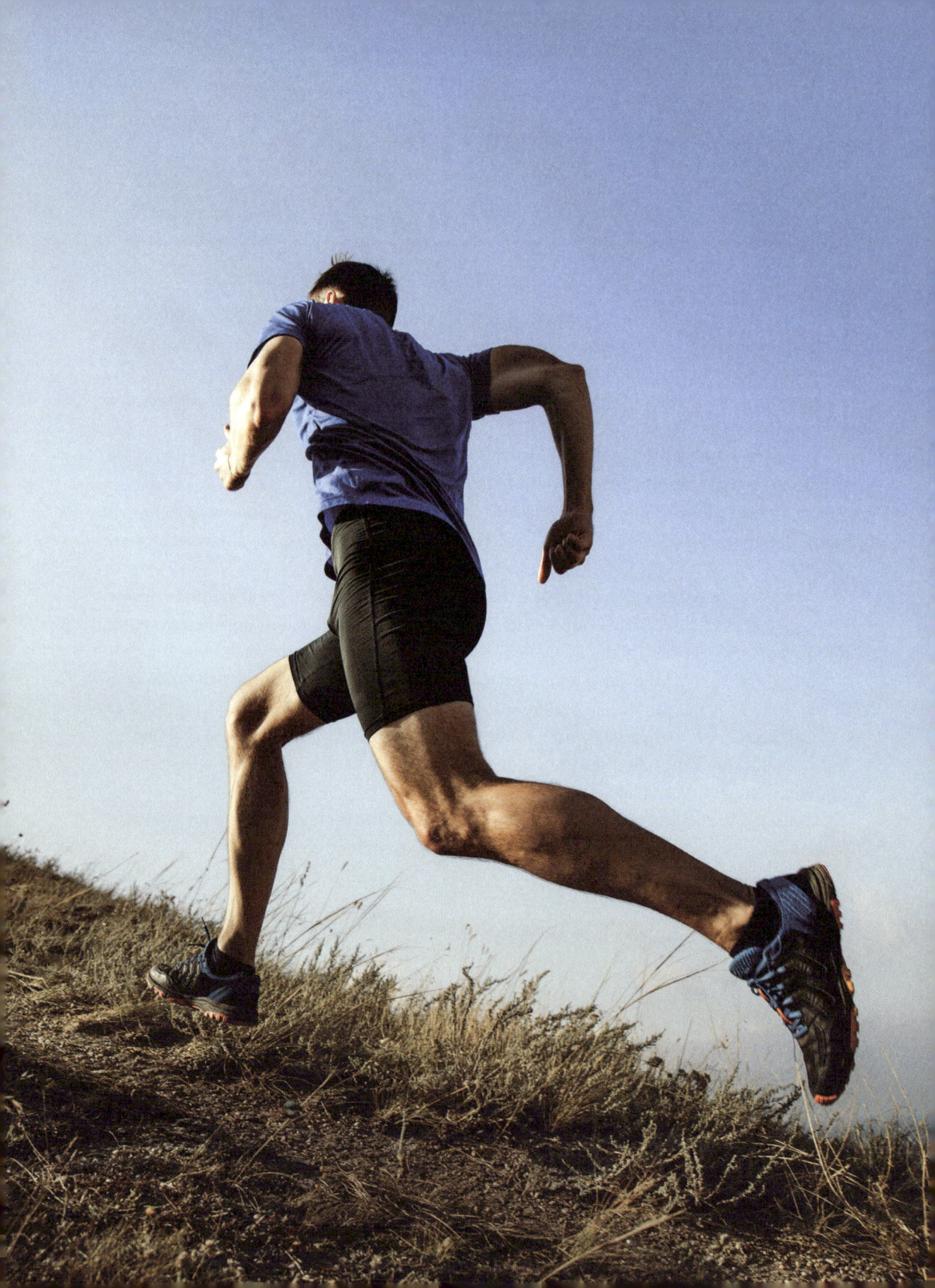

CHAPTER 1

Pilates is Perfect for Runners

So let me start by asking: **What kind of runner are you?**
To start, let's break down the top five types of runners and show you exactly how **Mat Pilates training** can be the not-so-secret weapon in everyone's training toolbox.

TYPES OF RUNNERS

The Casual Runner

Examples: Weekend joggers, running when convenient, fitness-focused runners, power walkers/joggers

Priorities: Injury prevention, general fitness, flexibility, core strength and mobility

How Pilates Helps: You don't need to be doing strict training for a race to reap the big benefits. Pilates trains your body to stay balanced, helps correct poor running habits (like overstriding, insufficient breathing or shoulder slouching), and ensures that you are engaging your core—not just pounding the pavement with your quads. It's the perfect way to feel stronger, smoother, more confident on your runs and recover faster. It also makes the runs more enjoyable. FYI—the author falls under the power walker/jogger category.

The Distance Runner

Examples: Marathoners, half-marathoners, long distance trail runners, ultramarathoners, kings and queens of cardio

Priorities: Endurance, longevity in your joints, efficient movement patterns, focus, adequate breath support

How Pilates Helps: Long-distance running can wear down your joints and lead to repetitive and overuse strain injuries. Pilates strengthens your deep core muscles, improves posture, and improves breath control—all of which add up to longer runs with less fatigue and better form. Plus, those delicious Pilates stretches are pure gold for tight hip flexors and hamstrings. What I say to my clients who love to go the distance is, "Strong core + pliable body = more miles with less wear and tear."

The Sprinter

Examples: Fast-twitch legends, track stars, powerful burst beasts

Priorities: Explosive speed, core strength, precise technique, reaction time

How Pilates Helps: Sprinters don't just run—they explode. And that explosive power? It comes from a rock-solid (core) foundation. Pilates gives you **explosive glute power, powerful hip mobility, and precision balance**. It teaches your body to move as one sleek, powerful unit. You'll rocket down that track with control, precision, and zero wasted movement. Bonus: your hamstrings will thank you. Perhaps they will send a Christmas card.

The Trail Runner

Examples: Nature ninjas, mountain climbers, rock-hopping heroes

Priorities: Core stability for uneven terrain, laser focus, special body awareness (proprioception)

How Pilates Helps: Trail runners like to live on the wild side. I know because I trail ran often when living in the Colorado mountains. It was always a challenge with the uneven terrain, random hikers, mountain bikers, fallen limbs and wild animals. Ever changing terrain? Mud? Hills? Elk? No problem! Pilates gives you **superhuman balance, ankle stability, and sharpened reflexes**. It fine-tunes your body awareness so you can leap logs and dodge roots like some kind of trail ninja. And deep core strength? It keeps your spine supported when the trail turns wildly unpredictable. Run strong, breathe deeper, and flow through the beautiful nature.

The Returning Runner

Examples: Making a comeback or taking those first strides as a beginner (Injured, recovering, rebuilding yourself back into a running phenom)

Priorities: Rebuilding your body from the inside out, gentle mobility and core strength, positive outlook, hope and encouragement

How Pilates Helps: Whether you're just starting out, you've been injured, burned out, or just need a break from the madness, Pilates is your **coach for both your first stab at running or your big comeback**. It builds you up from the inside out—core first, movement second, excitement third—so you don't just return, you return **stronger and better**. Gentle on the joints, focused on precision, and completely customizable, Pilates helps fix the imbalances and weaknesses that slowed you down in the first place. Control. Strength. Your comeback is complete. Remember: every great runner had to take those first few steps. We all do. Thank you Pilates for helping light the way!

No matter how you run, where you run, or why you run—**Pilates will make you a better runner**. Period. Core strength, flexibility, balance, breath—it's all in there, waiting to turn you into a well-oiled running machine. I've trained tens of thousands of diverse runners from all over the globe in Pilates and am constantly astounded at how powerfully they improve in just a short amount of time. So, get ready to roll out your mat, fire up those abs, and power up that stride!

BENEFITS OF PILATES FOR RUNNERS

Full disclosure: I'm not a "runner's runner," but hear me out.

When I agreed to write this book, I decided to lace up and take the *Pilates for Runners* journey right alongside you. Nearly every morning, I roll out of bed, chug a glass of water, and head straight into a hilly, curvy, lung-burning jog around my Tennessee neighborhood. And let me tell you—those hills mean serious business.

Now, I've always been more of a power walker by nature, but I wanted to put this powerful Pilates + running fusion to the ultimate test. So, I made a deal with myself: jog daily, practice Pilates daily, and see what happens. Most days, I follow up my run with 10–20 minutes of solo mat Pilates (yep, just Coach Vigue coaching…Coach Vigue. We can talk for hours about Pilates, running, film and opera), along with teaching live classes and filming online workouts for awesome people like you.

I've been practicing Pilates since 2005—but the running part—that became a real consistent habit in January 2025. I recorded a lot of that whole journey. I kept a journal of how my runs felt, what changed, what improved, what surprised me, and how Pilates played the leading role.

Here are a few summaries from that log:

Less Fatigue

I was running up the hills with more ease and the increased control over my strides and posture was very clear. The hills sucked at first, but after only a few days I was rather enjoying them and would return to the bottom and run up a few extra times feeling less winded and more triumphant. I walked on the side road in between and raised my arms in triumph like Rocky.

More Energy

I'm 51 not 20, so rolling out of bed, drinking a cup or two of water and heading outside to run in chilly Tennessee winter weather is not the most appealing. For most people it would be, "No way, are you nuts? Take more time to wake up and do a casual stroll around the neighborhood, Sean."

After a week of this training I was out the door like a rocket, ready to have some fun and build on what I accomplished the day before. It sounds strange, but I enjoy the hills the most and my energy levels increase in real time when I'm jogging up them. I have more energy reserves when I want to add on extra clicks (running terminology) and I don't really get that winded anymore. My mind is excited to move and see what improvements I've made.

Better Body Awareness

At first my shoulders, neck and head would feel uncomfortable. I was holding my body out of alignment with my head looking up too far, chin not slightly tucked, shoulders clenched and lifting up towards my ears and my head rang (hurt) because my strides were not smooth. I was running on heavy feet trying to find a smooth stride.

Regular running and Pilates practice made me very aware of how I was moving, how heavy I was landing my feet and the inefficient way I was using my body. Too much swinging of the arms was throwing me off balance and using up my precious energy stores. The more Pilates exercises I added each day, the more aware I was of how my body was moving through space and that translated to smoother, more efficient running strides.

Smoother Strides

It's wild, but strengthening my deep core muscles with the power of Pilates makes me run smoother. The core acts as a shock absorber and a strong flexible one really absorbs the repetitive bouncing of the feet striking the ground. When the core is weak, I can REALLY feel each individual foot strike and I don't like it. The extra core power also helps me stand taller, feel more confident and adjust my posture. The confidence part is key to getting me out on these runs consistently. I knew I could do it, so I kept "doing it." Having a strong, balanced and flexible core is a win-win for everything in life, not just running.

Looking Forward to Running

At first, I was rather hesitant. I hadn't gone on a technical run in many years. I started to improve when my mind began celebrating the runs I successfully completed and actually looking forward to the next one. It's exciting! I'm not out to do an intense run each day for many miles but my 30 minute sojourns really hit the spot, and I look forward to each one—even when it's snowing.

More Capable

With my new improved runs, I felt more capable in other aspects of my life i.e. yoga, teaching, family life, sports, strength training and more. Expanding my running abilities made me feel like I was back in junior high wrestling practice where we ran *every* practice up and down stairs, down hallways, across fields, and on the track. Knowing I'm improving so many aspects of my daily life makes me feel great!

Validation

I feel validated as I've been teaching Pilates and its many benefits for almost 20 years in live classes, videos, conferences, personal training, books and articles. It's inspiring to experience it in person and be able to add more layers to my teaching—I've lived it in many ways, this adds another facet to my teaching and my life.

Every single part of my running has improved thanks to Pilates. We're talking smoother strides, stronger core, better posture, and muscles that operate like a well-oiled Pilates machine. The secret? A hearty, diverse mix of Pilates exercises—yes, the very ones you'll find in this book—that keep me flexible, balanced, powerful, and ready for anything. A few exercises pack a mighty punch.

10 REASONS WHY RUNNERS WHO SKIP PILATES ARE MISSING OUT

Pilates is the runner's secret weapon. Say it with me again. Now jot it down on a sticky note and slap it on your water bottle. Use it as your mantra daily and, especially, when your runs are feeling hard and never ending. Whether you're a seasoned marathoner, a casual jogger, or thinking, "Maybe I'll give this running thing a try," this book has your name written all over it. Here's the truth: everyone runs. Young, old, fast, slow, smooth, rusty, clunky, uphill, downhill, on muddy trails—we've all done it. And no matter how or why you run, Pilates can help you run better.

This book is all about **Mat Pilates training**—a full-body, bodyweight-only program designed to build strength, boost mobility, and punch your core like never before. We'll get into the eight foundational principles of Pilates in Chapter 2, but here's the CliffsNotes version: Mat Pilates is your ticket to a limber, strong, flexible body that moves with breath, precision, and power. No equipment, no excuses—you can do this style of training *anywhere*, anytime, at any level. *And* it will help you do it all longer, stronger and better. It's completely accessible and immediately transforming.

I put together this list with you in mind. Every reason is important and essential. Every benefit is real. And every runner—yes, I'm speaking directly to YOU—needs Pilates in their arsenal.

Stronger, Balanced & More Flexible Core

Time for a crash course in your incredible core! Before we dive into the much anticipated Pilates moves, let's shine a spotlight on the muscles that make up your core. Yep, there's more to it than just training abs—so buckle up, because we're going in. I can't talk about Pilates without breaking down the powerhouse that drives it all: your core**.** Let's meet the muscles that make the magic happen!

The core muscles are made up of the abdominals, lower back, pelvic floor muscles and hip muscles. Here's a quick description of each so you can wow your friends in Trivial Pursuit:

The abdominals are made up of the rectus abdominis (the "six-pack" muscles), obliques (the sides of the abdomen), and the transverse abdominis (the deep muscle that wraps around the spine).

The lower back muscles include the erector spinae, the multifidus, the quadratus lumborum, the latissimus dorsi and other muscles along the spine that help support posture and movement.

The pelvic floor muscles are a group of muscles that form a "hammock" or "sling" at the base of the pelvis, providing support to the pelvic organs (including the bladder, uterus, and rectum) and playing a vital role in supporting core stability, controlling bladder and bowel functions, and improving sexual health. The pelvic muscles are composed of the levator ani, coccygeus, bulbospongiosus, ischiocavernosus and transverse perineal muscles. The pelvic floor works in coordination with the diaphragm, abdominals, and back muscles to form part of the body's core stability system. The pelvic floor muscles are essential in Pilates because they provide deep core and pelvis stability during movement. Engaging these muscles helps improve posture, balance, and overall control, which are key for running success.

The hip muscles include the hip flexors, glutes, and surrounding muscles that contribute to balance, smooth movement and stability. Strong, flexible and stable hips are a fundamental part of a runner's overall fitness and help promote increased speed, endurance, and overall running mechanics.

So, how does a strong core help create a faster, more efficient and overall better runner? Here's the list. Ready? Brace yourself—it's a lot of gold. This will also make perfect sense when you experience the Pilates exercises firsthand and feel the difference in your running.

First, it **helps keep your torso stable and supported,** which reduces the likelihood of slouching, bad posture or leaning forward during a run. Leaning forward severely cuts off your ability to breathe efficiently. This is particularly important for long runs, as poor posture can lead to fatigue and discomfort from your body constantly fighting to stay upright. Better posture and body alignment opens up deeper and more efficient inhales and exhales as well as increased endurance from the extra surge of energy. Not constantly fighting bad posture, opening up your breath and diaphragm (the primary muscle responsible for inhalation and exhalation) control will give you a huge jolt of free energy to be expended on better overall running technique.

Core muscles help **maintain a neutral spine alignment,** which is needed for efficient movement and strides. Poor alignment can lead to tremendous strain on muscles and joints, increasing the risk of injury and being sidelined over time.

A strong Pilates core **activates better control over your body's movement during running,** no matter the intensity or distance. It helps train the upper and lower body to propel forward with fluidity and coordination. Without a strong, balanced core, your arms and legs have trouble syncing up properly, which will lead to imbalances that can hamper your training.

You will experience **better efficiency and power** as your core plays a crucial role in the transfer of energy between the upper and lower body. While running, power is generated from the legs, and a strong core (center) efficiently transfers this energy up through the torso, creating a smoother, looser and more powerful stride. Again, that will increase your endurance, injury prevention (read on) and overall enjoyment of running. Smoother runs can also lead to a more satisfying runners high (the euphoric feeling runners may experience during or after a run).

And finally, by building proper posture and movement patterns, a strong core **reduces the strain and fatigue on other muscle groups,** which can lead to reduced soreness, tightness and discomfort after runs. Balanced core strength also helps reduce the impact (pounding) on joints, particularly the lower back, hips, and knees, helping runners recover more quickly and effectively.

Injury Prevention & Recovery

I've trained thousands of runners and have seen a multitude of injuries that keep them sidelined and frustrated. Runners are very susceptible to overuse injuries (shin splints, runner's knee, Achilles tendonitis, plantar fasciitis, muscle strains, stress fractures and IT band syndrome—more on these in a few paragraphs—to name a few) often caused by repetitive movements, muscle imbalances, insufficient blood flow, poor posture, and bad alignment. Pilates addresses these issues by strengthening the muscles, improving flexibility, and enhancing overall body awareness.

Doing Pilates exercises and workouts daily will help reverse these causes by building a strong core, restoring mobility into your muscles and building awareness of proper posture in all positions that translates to less time being sidelined with injuries.

Pilates exercises focus on smooth, controlled, low-impact movements to help runners recover faster by improving circulation, decreasing muscle tightness, and building muscle balance. This makes Pilates an excellent companion to your running program, helping runners (and all athletes) recover faster and more effectively after long runs or hard workouts.

Improved Flexibility

Pilates helps improve the flexibility (the ability to move your joints and muscles through a full range of motion without pain) of joints, which is essential for better runner performance. A higher level of flexibility reduces the risk of injuries such as those pesky muscle strains, tight hamstrings and calves, or IT band issues by allowing for a greater—and more confident— range of motion during each stride and heel strike.

Note: Pay special attention to the seated exercises in Chapter 3 for an extra dose of full body flexibility.

Pilates Fits Perfectly with the Runner's Schedule

Pilates will meet you exactly where you are—at home, on the road, training on a track or running the treadmill. Mat Pilates needs no equipment, only your bodyweight and you can create a workout perfectly tailored to your needs here and now. Flip ahead to Chapters 4–6 for 14 effective workouts for all your training needs.

Balanced Muscular Strength

Running really pounds the same muscle groups repeatedly. These include the core muscles (abdominals and low back), quads, hamstrings, calves, glutes, hip flexors and shins. Without relief these areas lose their elasticity, function and pliability. Pilates targets the whole body, ensuring all muscles are strengthened evenly, which will help correct muscle imbalances that might hinder running efficiency.

Enhances Stability & Balance

Runners are forced with each step to navigate always changing terrain, weather and people and objects around them. Pilates exercises boost proprioception (your personal sense of body position) and improve balance, which is essential for runners in preventing falls, exploring uneven terrain, and sustaining control and focus on longer or more difficult runs.

Greater Mind-Body Connection

Doing Pilates exercises requires total focus and concentration. This translates to helping runners cultivate better awareness of their body mechanics. The mind sees it and the body does it…or as Joseph Pilates put it, "Pilates is complete coordination of body, mind and spirit" and, "It's the mind itself which shapes the body." Pilates is your catalyst for not just drastically improved running technique and function but also building a stronger self in mind, body and spirit.

More Powerful & Efficient Breathing

Runners of all types require a steady supply of oxygen to fuel their muscles and body. Pilates encourages diaphragmatic or "deep belly" breathing, where the diaphragm (a large muscle beneath the lungs) is activated, causing deeper and more efficient breaths. Regular Pilates training teaches us to fully expand the lungs and use the diaphragm. This translates to runners increasing lung capacity and improving oxygen intake during short, medium and long runs, boosting endurance and stamina. Deep breathing also helps reduce stress, focus the mind and improve posture. I'm taking a deep breath right now.

Enhanced Endurance

Pilates is a fantastic way to increase muscular endurance, particularly because it focuses on building strength through controlled, precise movements with high repetitions and very low impact on the body. With this improved muscular endurance, runners are able to run longer distances with less fatigue. The increased blood flow and stronger heart function feed oxygen starved muscles during even the most challenging runs.

"Pilates is a Way of Life"

As Joseph Pilates once said, "The Pilates method teaches you to be in control of your body and not at its mercy."

I've been practicing and teaching Pilates for over 20 years, and I've *never* regretted a single workout. Not one. I've taught over 5,000 live classes and filmed twice as many online, and every (almost) single session has been a success. Why? Because Pilates delivers real results. Every. Single. Time.

During and after each class both my students and I feel the same incredible benefits: more energy, sharper focus, stronger muscles, better posture, boosted mood, and bodies that are more flexible, capable, and ready for anything. That's not just hype—it comes from solid experience. It's also what millions of my clients around the world have shared with me through in-person sessions, online workouts, and my books.

Pilates time is a special power time—a beautifully focused, unforgettable experience where the outside world melts away and your body stretches, strengthens, and transforms. The more you practice, the more you improve. I call it **progressive destabilization**: each workout challenges you a little more, forcing your body to adapt, stabilize, and get stronger in real time. It's functional, dynamic, and wildly effective.

And look, I know these are just words. Words don't do the sweating, breathing, or training for you. But they can get you to the mat—and once you're there, the words fade and the real magic begins. You move, you flow, and everything changes. You're in the Pilates zone!

So why am I telling you all this? Simple—to get you fired up for Chapter 3, where we dive headfirst into the delicious, transformational world of Pilates exercises and flowing routines that'll support every step of your running journey.

But before we jump in, let's take a quick look at something every runner needs to know: how to avoid injury during a run.

THE TOP 5 MOST COMMON RUNNING INJURIES

Thanks to its emphasis on both stability and mobility, Pilates is a huge asset in helping prevent injury and facilitate recovery. This is especially true for the most common types of injuries encountered by runners. Let's break it down!

Runner's Knee (Patellofemoral Pain Syndrome)

Runner's knee is characterized by pain around or under the kneecap, notably where it meets the lower end of the thighbone (femur). Causes include overuse of the knee joint from the repetitive pounding of running, muscular imbalances from weak, atrophied and tight muscles stemming from the thighs and hips and poor postural alignment of the kneecap, thighbone, ankle and foot.

How Pilates Helps: The strong, balanced core from Pilates will help stabilize your pelvis and legs while running, helping your knees in tracking properly over your feet. You will also maintain better alignment throughout your run and stronger hips which will prevent the inward collapse of the knee (valgus knee), which contributes to runner's knee.

Shin Splints (Medial Tibial Stress Syndrome)

Shin splints refers to pain along the shinbones (the tibia) which can be caused by the repetitive stress and overuse on the low part of the legs, wearing improper footwear which offers little or no support when running, running too much without appropriate rest, lack of a proper pre-running warm up, training on hard and uneven surfaces and poor posture and stride technique.

How Pilates Helps: A strong core can reduce the pressure and load on your legs to prevent overuse injuries, stretches the muscles around the Achilles tendon, shins and calves improving flexibility and decreasing tightness and correcting muscle imbalances, equalizing muscular strength and mobility through your legs and core to correct these imbalances.

Achilles Tendinitis

This is another overuse injury and it causes pain, inflammation and swelling in the Achilles tendon, which is the thick band of tissue connecting the calf muscle to the heel bone.

How Pilates Helps: Working and stretching the calves and hamstrings puts less strain on the tendon, better posture and alignment will help balance your weight evenly across the body, reducing excess weight on the tendon and Pilates is a very low impact exercise which places less stress on the body.

Here's a Coach Vigue tip: Grab a tennis or Lacrosse ball and massage it on the bottom of your feet. It will help massage the fascia and release tension but be cautious: the lacrosse ball can get pretty intense.

Plantar Fasciitis

Ouch! This can really be uncomfortable. Plantar fasciitis is a common condition in which the thick band that runs along the bottom of the foot from the heel to the toes becomes inflamed. The foot can become very tender and swell or even painful as weight is placed on the feet.

How Pilates Helps: By now, you understand how Pilates is a sort of cure-all for your running woes. Here are a few reasons why Pilates will help with that pesky and performance sidelining Plantar fasciitis: it stretches and releases tight calves and hamstrings which add to the tension on the plantar fascia; it improves flexibility in the foot and ankle area; and it promotes full body balance and stability which pulls unnecessary weight off the feet. Pilates exercises are low impact and can be performed when recovering from a bout of PF and the big P helps correct muscle imbalances which can be linked to that pesky discomfort on the bottom of your feet.

Remember my Coach Vigue tip? It pulls double duty here. Use a tennis or lacrosse ball to massage the bottom of your feet. It will help release the fascia and promote blood flow.

IT Band Syndrome (Iliotibial Band Syndrome)

This is basically another overuse injury (running is very repetitive, it seems) that causes pain on the outside of the knee radiating from the IT band, a thick tendon that runs along the outside of the thigh from the hip to the knee. The tendon becomes swollen and tender to the touch. It can also be quite painful and discouraging as any movement in the knee is difficult.

How Pilates Helps: Pilates corrects muscle imbalances and improves alignment in the hips and pelvis, reducing tension on the IT band. Pilates also strengthens key stabilizing muscles like the glutes and core, which support correct leg tracking during movement.

INTEGRATING PILATES INTO YOUR RUNNING SCHEDULE

Pilates and running are as easy to integrate as peanut butter and jelly (or jam—jam is better) and much less messy. It has been my goal as a fitness instructor for 20+ years to make world class health and fitness as accessible and easy to add to your busy schedule as possible. Once married together and practiced daily it becomes a habit and then you can't function without it. You can try but your running and life will suffer tremendously. I speak from experience. Without daily movement and exercise I get irritable, stiff and moody. Just ask my wife.

Here's ten easy ways to incorporate Pilates into your daily schedule without missing a beat. The greatest gym membership is your body—it's with you 24/7, just waiting to be activated. So, these Pilates mat exercises will upload into your daily routine with ease.

Practice first thing in the morning.

This will wake your body up gently, get your breathwork moving, set an amazing tone of fluid movement for the day and will get you out of bed (or off the floor) with a fired up core which will reinforce good posture all day.

Include a pre-run warm-up to fire up your body.

Use dynamic Pilates moves like the 100, roll ups, or single straight leg stretch to gently warm up the hips, spine, and hamstrings before your run. Or, for a post-run Pilates cooldown, ditch the static stretching and add saws, lying spinal twists, hamstring stretches with breath (rowing), or gentle spinal articulation to restore length, release and mobility.

Work in Pilates during breaks in your day.

Re-energize your mind and body during breaks at your desk, home, the park and even practice. Pilates is definitely an energizing practice that will help you avoid fatigue and energy dips throughout the day.

Incorporate Pilates into your strength training workouts.

On cross-training days, mix Pilates exercises into your strength routine. Use it as your warm-up, finisher, replace one gym day with a full Pilates session or just drop down and do Pilates in between sets. That's what I do. Carry a mat with you around the gym and lay it down next to the squat rack, bench press and weight rack. Do a set, fire up with some Pilates and jump right back into strength training with more energy, core power and precision. Avoid weights falling on your head.

Activate your core before speed & hill workouts.

Before high-stress runs, do a few minutes of core, hip and glute activation (planks, side leg, Saw, bridges). This wakes and fires up key postural stabilizers so you'll run more efficiently with greater speed and precision.

Cultivate a bedtime Pilates routine to relax.

Ditch the phone unless you're doing my YouTube workouts or streaming while hunched over for 10–15 minutes of slow, relaxing Pilates stretches—how about spine twists, roll downs, and deep breaths. It's a fantastic way to develop a wind down and recovery routine that will improve your sleep consistency.

Practice while watching TV or listening to music.

Every night when the house is asleep I go downstairs and roll onto the floor to write, study and, of course, to do my evening Pilates and flexibility routines. I'm a night owl and yearn to do my best work between 9 pm and 1 am. My special time. I need just a little bit of space to create a full Pilates core centered workout which I never repeat. I go to bed stronger, leaner, more flexible and ready for a good eight hours of deep sleep…hopefully.

Take classes at your local gym or Pilates studio.

Find an excellent instructor who knows how to put together and cue effective Pilates workouts or work one-on-one with a trainer. Taking your Pilates practice into a class or one-on-one setting will enhance the training from this book!

If they have Pilates Reformer classes, take full advantage.

Reformer classes are fantastic because the spring resistance and sliding carriage add intensity, control, and support to movements, helping build strength, flexibility, and alignment all at once. They're also super effective for targeting smaller stabilizing muscles that are often missed in traditional workouts, hence hitting the runner where they most need help.

Train with me online!

What a shameless plug! Well, my YouTube videos are very diverse and accessible for all the runner's needs. Beginner, Intermediate, advanced, runner focused and more—I have them. Better yet, do my Pilates for Runners series created specifically for this book...and YOU.

With all that out of the way, let's get started—and where better than with the basics!

5 EASY WAYS TO INTEGRATE PILATES INTO YOUR RUNNING ROUTINE

And that's *without* overloading your schedule—perfect for keeping your body balanced, injury-free, and strong.

1. PRE-RUN ACTIVATION (5–10 mins)

Do a quick mat-based warm-up to activate your core, glutes, and hips. Think bridges, toe taps, and spinal articulations to prep your body for impact.

2. POST-RUN RECOVERY FLOW (10–15 mins)

Use Pilates stretches like the saw, spine stretch, and hip openers to release tight muscles and enhance mobility after runs.

3. ONE FULL MAT SESSION WEEKLY (30–45 mins)

Schedule one focused mat Pilates session per week to build core strength, improve alignment, and work on imbalances. Treat it like your cross-training day!

4. CORE WORK ON REST DAYS (10–20 mins)

Keep it simple: a short core-focused Pilates flow on your non-running days keeps your posture sharp and your back happy.

5. REPLACE ONE EASY RUN WITH PILATES (1/month)

Once in a while, swap an easy jog for a low-impact, high-reward Pilates class—your joints and muscles will thank you.

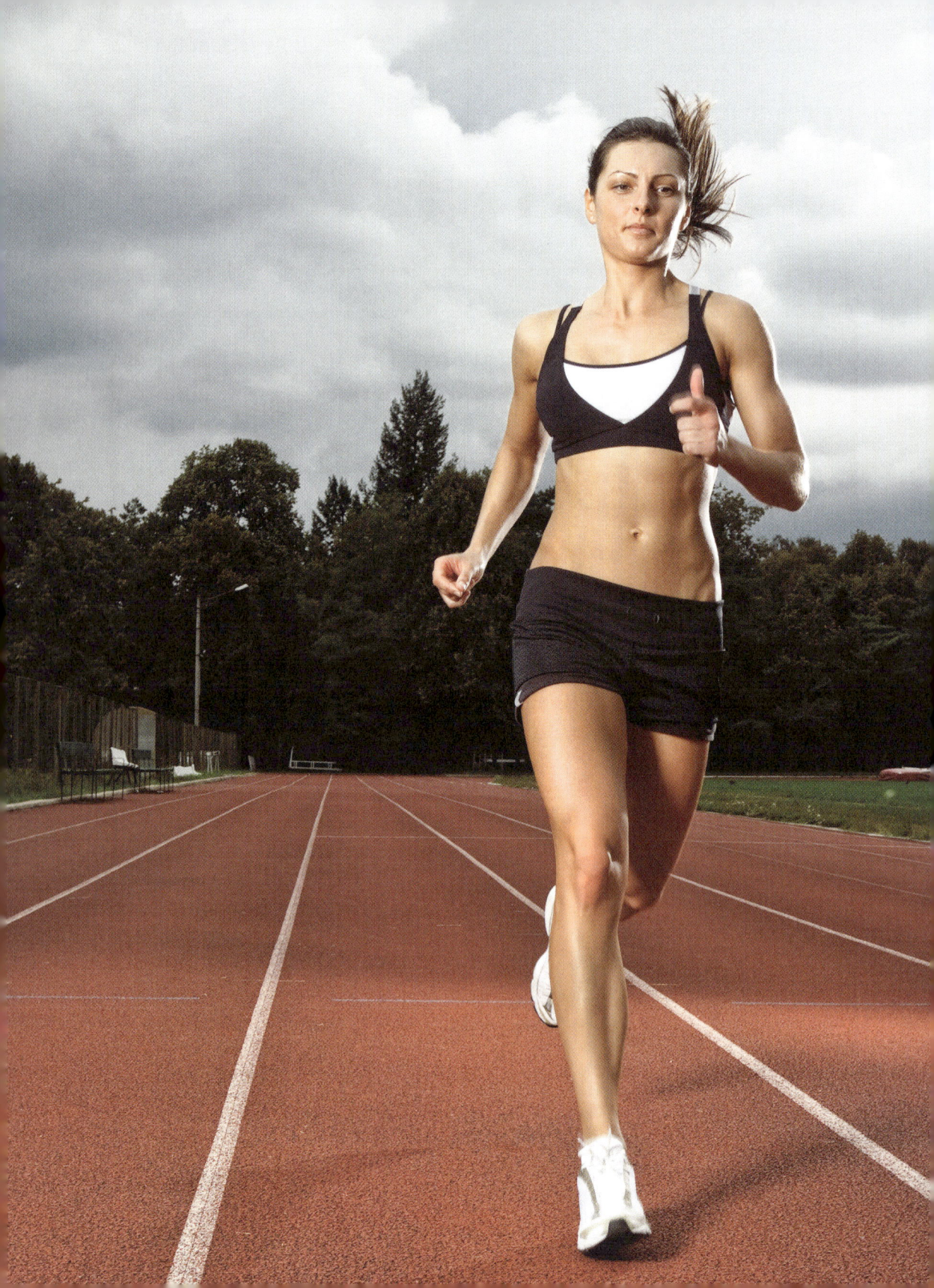

CHAPTER 2

The Basics of Pilates Mat Training

I know you can almost *hear* those Pilates exercises calling to you from just over the hill up ahead—so let's discuss why the method used in this book, Pilates Mat, is such a powerful, performance boosting weapon for runners like you. We'll start by diving into the legendary **Eight Principles of Pilates**, the secret ingredients that take your training from average to unstoppable.

First, a quick refresher: the Pilates method featured in this book is **Mat Pilates**—the purest form of Pilates. This means no weights, no machines, no excuses—just your bodyweight, a mat, some comfy clothes, and a little space where you can focus and flow. It's incredibly efficient, completely adaptable, and fits into any runner's schedule—whether you're sprinting at sunrise or going for a jog after work.

Mat Pilates is the bread and butter of the Pilates world. It's raw, real, and ridiculously effective. You can do it anywhere—the beach, the gym, your living room, a mountain top, or even backstage at a theater (been there! West Side Story is a very strenuous show). It uses gravity and your own body to build strength, sculpt muscle, and boost flexibility. Abs? Burning. Glutes? Activated. Hamstrings? Long and strong. You're also mastering control, alignment, and breath—no fancy, clunky machines required. Just you and the mat, working in sweet, sweaty harmony. Someone put that last sentence on a t-shirt!

I've taught over **5,000 Pilates Mat classes** in places like Walt Disney World, Florida Hospital, dance studios, town halls, and national fitness conferences. And for every class I've taught live, I've filmed three times as many for my global online audience of millions who can't get enough of this *total-body* powerhouse method.

I've also spread the Pilates love on hundreds of podcasts, written nine books and even popped up in films and TV showing how Pilates transforms bodies even for folks like Juliette

Binoche and Jeff Goldblum (yep, that actually happened—and will again and again). When I was a professional singer/actor performing around the country in live theater I figured I'd appear on film and television but it's been my long and rewarding career in the world of fitness that ended up putting me on the big screen.

So why am I telling you all this? Because before we dive headfirst into the workouts, you've got to understand the Eight Pilates Principles—your mental and physical blueprint for doing Pilates safely, effectively, and with maximum results. These aren't just rules—they're the nucleus of the practice. When you embrace these, you don't just *do* Pilates…you *live* it. You become the Pilates and Pilates never leaves.

Let's break them down—why they matter, and how they'll help you run stronger, recover faster, and move like a well-oiled machine.

CONCENTRATION

Pilates effectiveness thrives on mental presence and 100 percent focus on each breath, moment and movement. Concentration ensures proper form and helps you connect deeply with the movements and rhythms of your body. It turns exercise into a mindful (albeit enjoyable) practice, providing results and reducing the risk of injury. Pilates demands your full attention and if your concentration drifts so will the exercises, and so will the benefits. Every movement has a purpose. There are no accidents in Pilates, just intentions.

CONTROL

Every movement in Pilates is done with precise intention and control—avoid rushing, jerking, or momentum. "Keep it smooth," I always say. This builds effective strength and stability while training the mind and body to move more efficiently. Control also keeps those smaller neglected stabilizing muscles engaged and firing. If you can't control the movement, no benefits shall be had. A quote that I come back to frequently is, "Range is for the ego, control is for the soul."

CENTERING

Every movement comes from your "powerhouse"—the core muscles around your abdomen, lower back, hips, and glutes. Centering helps develop strength, awareness and support in this area, improving posture and balance. It's the dominant grounding force for the rest of your body. Every movement first originates in your core. Keep your mind's eye always focused on that core.

PRECISION

In Pilates I always say it is quality over quantity. Every movement has a purpose; there are no accidents. Pilates demands absolute exactness in movement—even the smallest adjustments can make a huge difference. Precision guarantees that you are targeting the correct muscles and avoiding compensation patterns that favor certain areas that lead to imbalance. The more precision you demand from your Pilates workouts, the more improvement you'll witness when pounding the pavement.

BREATH

As my dear college voice teacher Mr. Johnson used to say, "Everything begins with a breath" As each day passes, his words have a greater impact, especially in my Pilates practice…and when singing Puccini. Breathing in Pilates is synched with movement and enhances focus and oxygen utilization. It fires up core engagement and helps maintain rhythm and control. Focused breathwork also calms the nervous system and improves the mind-body connection. Your breathing and lungs are like any muscle and need to be consistently worked to become stronger.

FLOW

Flow, flow, flow. It's all flow. When my life isn't in a state of flow, I feel stagnant, incomplete and ineffective. The exercises in Pilates are smooth, continuous, and graceful—not stiff or rigid. Flow invites fluid exercise transitions and creates dynamic and connected workouts. The emphasis on flow is what makes Pilates feel smooth and efficient. Life in general feels better with flow. Flow in all things and watch it improve your running mechanics.

ALIGNMENT

If it ain't aligned, it ain't going to work properly. Proper alignment is the foundation of effective and safe movement, especially running. When your spine, pelvis, and limbs are in the correct position, you build balanced strength and avoid unnecessary strain during your runs. Pilates teaches runners to recognize and correct imbalances in real time, becoming a more efficient manner. This awareness carries into any intensity of running and helps you run longer, faster and with more ease.

INTEGRATION

Integration brings everything together: mind, body, breath, and powerful running movement. Every Pilates exercise combines the other seven principles into a strong and effective unified whole. When fully integrated, Pilates becomes more than just exercise; it becomes a practice of total body awareness, movement and harmony. This translates into better and more enjoyable runs, no matter the distance, terrain or intensity. It's what makes Pilates feel so balanced and intentional…and your runs will feel the same way.

Here's the deal: once you really understand and apply these Pilates principles, you'll see it's so much more than just another fad workout—it becomes a precision tool for runners. We're talking strength, flexibility, mental sharpness…all wrapped up in one powerful training discipline. There's this beautiful, unpredictable madness of it all—and once Pilates becomes part of your daily training habit that precision attitude starts to click. You'll feel it. You'll own it. You'll never look back.

HOW TO USE THIS BOOK

I wrote this book with one mission: **to help runners of all ages, levels, and styles easily and effortlessly add Mat Pilates into their training and unlock a bonanza of benefits.** That's it. Simple. No fluff. No hidden agenda. My goal is to get you moving, because once you start moving all the good stuff starts—better performance, smoother strides, fewer injuries, stronger muscles, sharper focus…the list goes on. It all "clicks."

This book is your training partner—take it anywhere, flip to any page, and stay inspired, active, connected to your practice and conquer your runs. Which brings us to the two main ways I recommend using this book in your daily life. (Of course, feel free to make Pilates training your own—as long as your form and precision are rock solid!) You know better than anyone how to plan and execute your training schedule.

STEP 1. MASTER THE INDIVIDUAL EXERCISES

Pick a move, practice it, and feel how it supports and influences your running. Perhaps you're having issues with a particular body part or area. Find your favorites—the ones that give you the biggest return for your time and energy. Honestly, every single exercise in this book is designed to level up and improve not just your running, but your overall movement, control, and flow

STEP 2. TACKLE THE WORKOUTS

Choose a workout—five of them, all of them, whatever feels right. Here's the only rule: **don't rush it.** Practice each exercise until your form is so precise you can teach it, then (and only then) perform the full workout, linking each move together with breath and flow. Rinse and repeat as often as you like—you'll get stronger, more focused, and more fluid every single time.

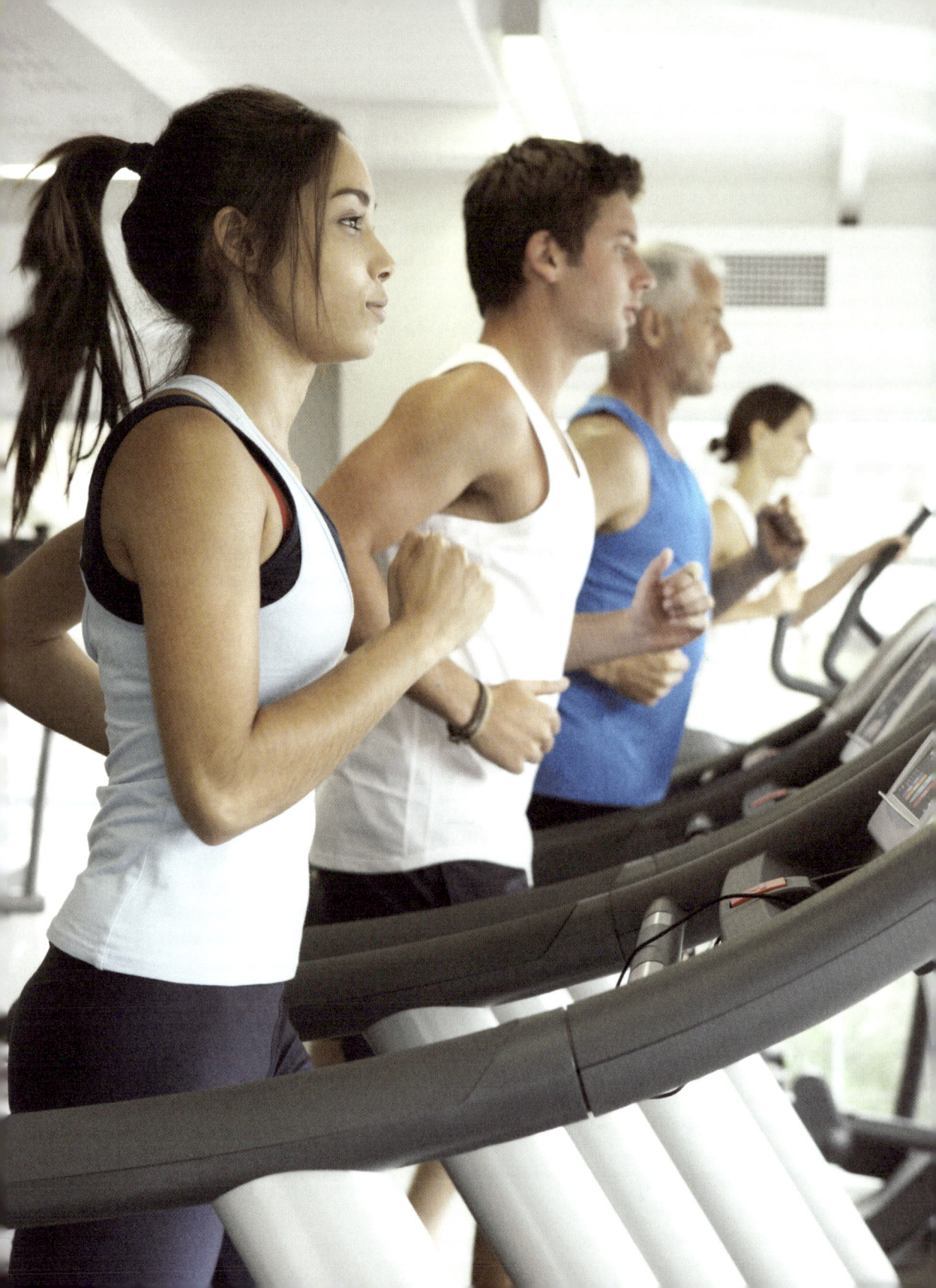

CHAPTER 3

The Exercises

Alright, runners—it's go time. We've stretched, breathed, and talked about the magic of Pilates, but now we're hitting and slicing the meat and potatoes of this book—the part where transformation actually occurs.

We could chat all day about how Pilates helps you run stronger, recover faster, and move like a superhero—but let's be honest: nothing changes until you roll out your mat, take a deep breath (and keep breathing!), and start moving. That's when the real magic kicks in.

What you're about to dive into are my **Top 40 Pilates Mat Exercises for Runners**—plus **10 incredible yoga stretches** to boost flexibility, mobility, and recovery. This is your complete toolkit to level up your speed, form, endurance, injury prevention, and most importantly— your joy in movement. If you don't love it you're bound to give it up quickly.

Here's the deal: every single exercise is a mini-workout on its own. Focus deeply. Move with control. Breathe with purpose. Let each rep be packed with precision. We're not cranking out endless reps under my watch—we're going for quality over quantity to squeeze every drop of strength, flexibility, and power from each delicious move.

Enough talk. No more words, runners—it's time to MOVE!

A QUICK WORD ON PILATES BREATHING

Breath is everything in Pilates. Inhale through your nose, exhale through your mouth—smooth, steady, and controlled. Think of it like this: each inhale drowns your muscles with fresh, energizing oxygen. Each exhale wrings out your lungs like a wet washcloth, emptying every last drop. I always visualize my muscles soaking in that clean, fresh air and then purging every ounce of stale breath from my lungs.

Mastering your breathing will supercharge your energy, sharpen your focus, and keep you feeling strong and centered, on the mat and on the run.

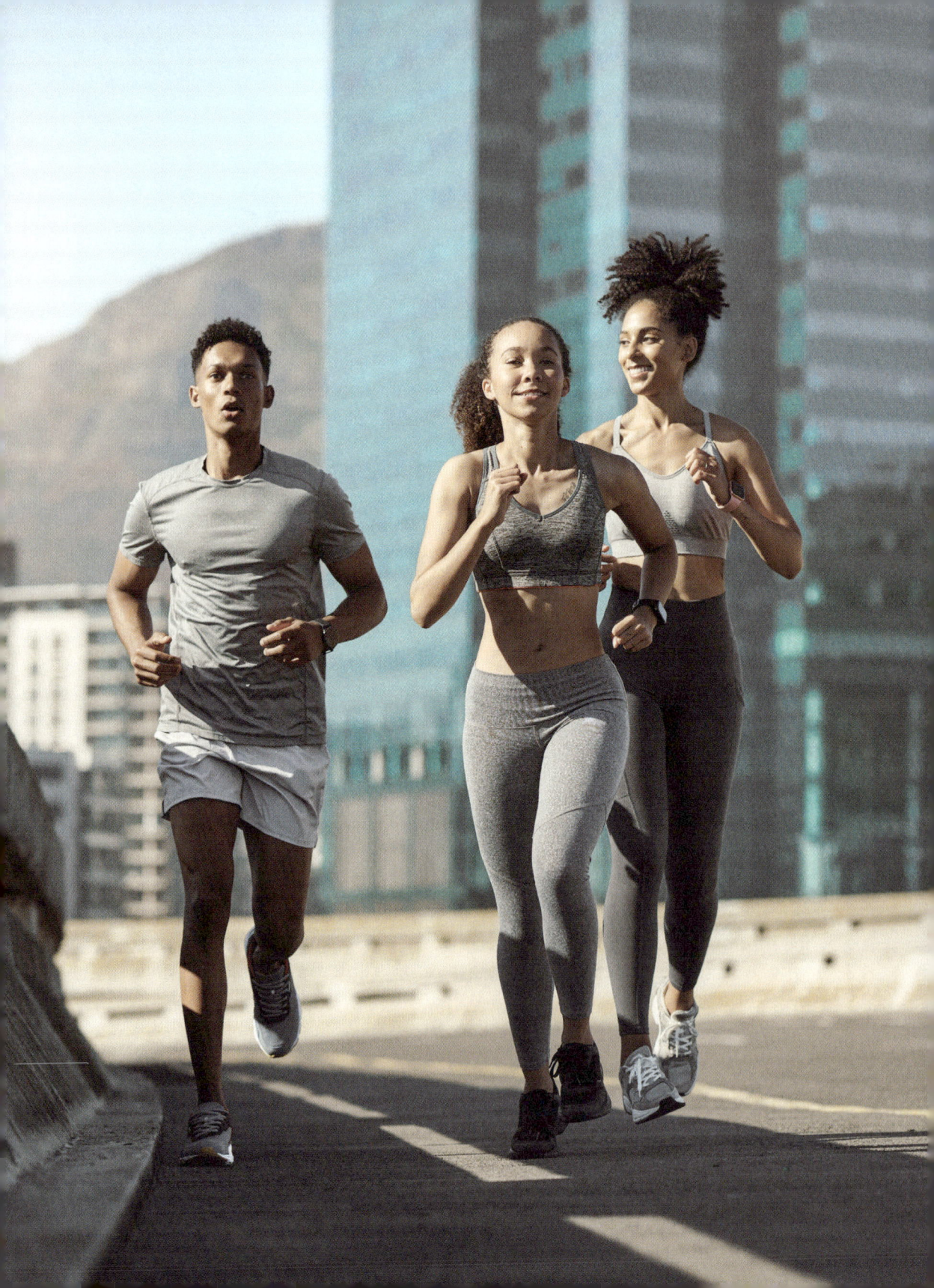

The Top 10 Pilates Mat Exercises for Runners

Build a strong foundation for efficient, injury-free running with these essential mat moves.

THE SAW

AREAS TARGETED: Core, hamstrings and calves

This one has it all: hip and hamstring flexibility, back mobility and core power.

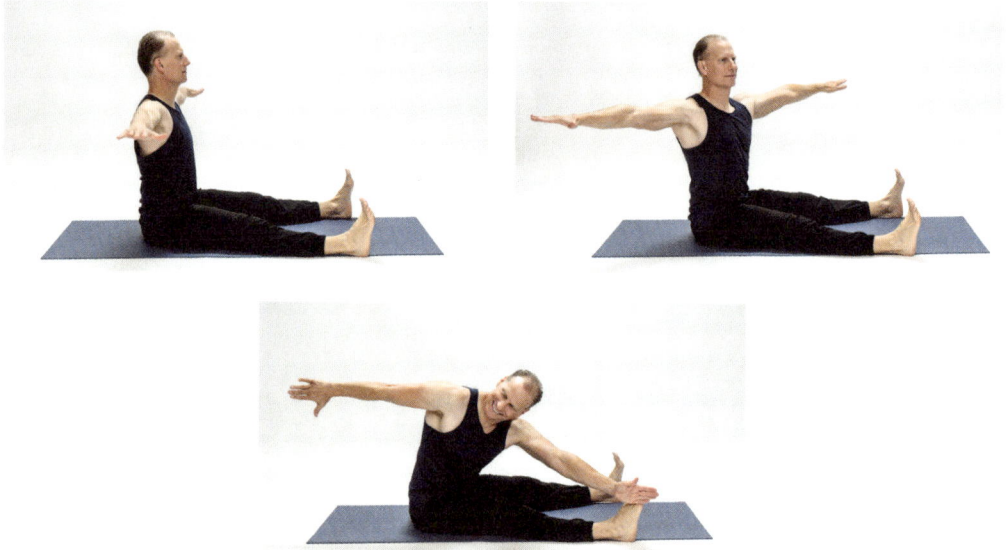

1. Sit tall with your arms side to side and open your legs so your heels are on the edges of the mat. Draw your toes towards you.

2. Inhale and twist to the right from the waist. Stay tall in your posture.

3. Exhale twice as you hinge forward and pulse your left pinky finger across your right pinky toe. Slice the toe with your finger! Do two pulses connected to the breath. Turn your head to look at your right arm. Inhale and return tall to the center and flow to the other side. Do 5 pulses on each side.

Key Points

- The Saw has the honor of twisting and stretching at the same time, which has the effect of "wringing" out your lungs.

- You have an opportunity to master the Pilates breathing technique with this exercise. The inhales help lift your upper body and the exhales assist in lengthening up and over the leg. Let the second breath on the pulse completely empty the lungs of air.

- The arms are always extended, straight and reaching in opposite directions.

SPINE STRETCH

AREAS TARGETED: Abdominals, calves, hamstrings and back

Stretch your spine and back muscles while hitting your hamstrings, hips and core.

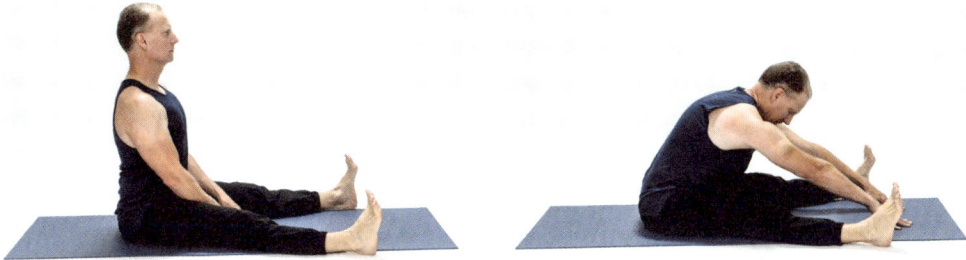

1. From a seated position, extend and open your legs so your heels are on the edges of the mat and your knees are rotated towards the sky. Draw your toes towards you and sit up tall with your shoulders back and down, chest open and chin slightly tucked. Inhale.

2. Exhale, chin to your chest, and place your fingertips on the ground. Hinge forward (into a C-curve) to the end of your range of motion.

3. Inhale and return to the starting position as if you were imprinting your spine against a wall behind you, one vertebra at a time. Repeat 5–8 times.

Key Points

- When hinging forward, imagine lifting your abdominals up and over a beach ball. This visual will reinforce moving your abs up and in towards the spine. Vacuum out the breath on the exhale. Squeeze out every drop.

- If cramping in the leg occurs, relax and wiggle your ankles and feet.

- Imagine someone pulling you forward from your hands to ensure maximum stretch and spinal articulation in the spine and back. Press the backs of your knees down to ignite the hamstrings and calves in a stretch for the ages.

■ SINGLE STRAIGHT LEG STRETCH

AREAS TARGETED: Core, hamstrings and low back

Strengthen your core, stretch the hamstrings, and teach your body to move with control, breath, and the grace of a cheetah sprinting across the plains!

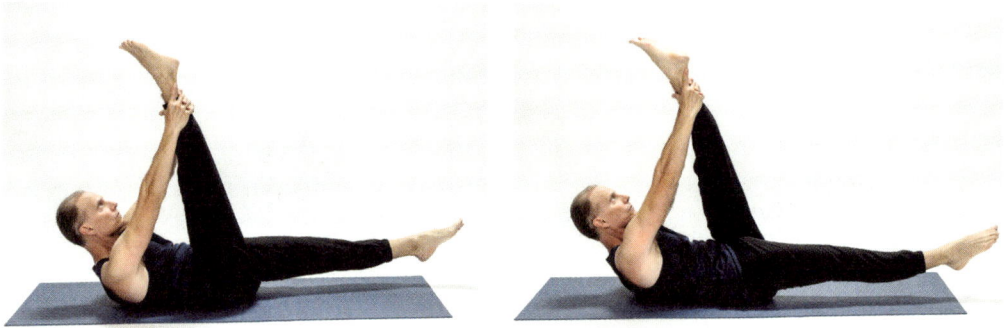

1. Lying on your back, extend your right leg to the ceiling and lengthen your left leg in front of you off the mat. Peel your head and shoulders off the mat while gently grabbing your right ankle or calf. Exhale twice as you pulse the leg towards you twice and contract the abdominals.

2. Inhale and switch (scissors) the legs and grasp the left leg for two pulses with the breath. Stabilize against the movement of the legs. Perform 5–10 repetitions.

Key Points

- This exercise moves at a brisk pace with quick changes of leg direction. Infuse that movement with breath and work on having zero strain in your core. Feel the lungs working with each exhale.

- Add an extra chest lift as you bring your leg towards you for a deeper contraction. Think of delivering your nose to the knee.

- Keep your spine flat on the mat during the duration of the movement and your elbows facing outward for more room to move.

FOREARM PLANK

AREAS TARGETED: Core, shoulders and arms

Fire up your body from the center outward and improve your focus, posture and stability.

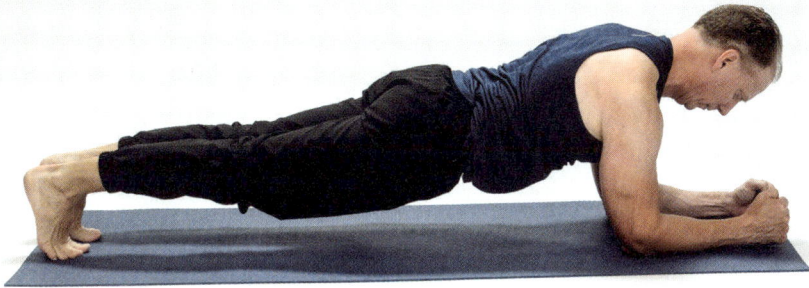

1. Move into plank position with your forearms on the ground, elbows under your shoulders, fingers laced together and heels pressing back behind you.

2. Draw your shoulders back and breathe steadily. Flex your abs as you exhale.

3. Hold for 10–20 breaths and stabilize your core.

Key Points

- Keep the back of your neck long with a slight chin tuck.
- You can add some serious spice to the plank by extending one arm forward at a time.

CRISS CROSS

AREAS TARGETED: Core (especially the obliques)

When performed with proper form, your abs will never be stronger.

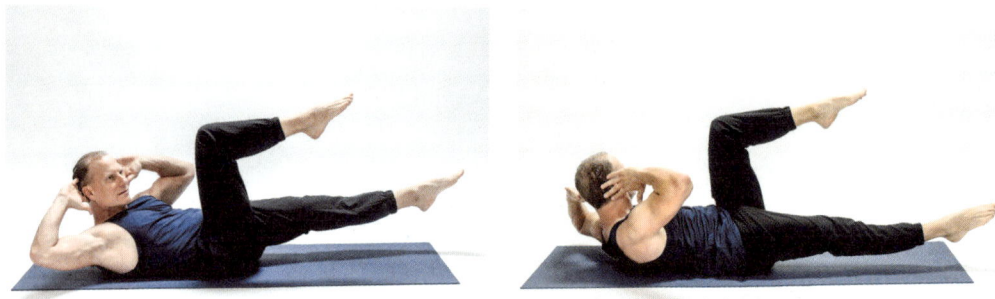

1. Lying on your back, place your fingers lightly on the back of your head so they are not touching. Your elbows should be relaxed to the sides. Draw your right knee towards you at a 90-degree angle and extend your left leg so it's slightly off the floor. With an exhale, bring your head, neck and shoulders off the mat, lifting your chest towards your right knee, creating a twist.

2. Inhale as you switch the legs and exhale as you activate the abdominals to bring the chest towards the left knee. Keep your elbows relaxed and out to the sides. Repeat 10–20 times.

Key Points

- Never, never, never bring your elbow to the opposite knee. I see this done all the time and it drives me crazy because it pulls the emphasis out of the core and places it on reaching an elbow to a knee. This torques the neck, causing undue strain and pressure. So don't do it!

- Avoid dipping your upper body in the center while moving side to side. This disengages the core and pushes into your lower back. Keep your upper body lifted through the entire exercise.

- Keep the thigh on your bent leg pointed upward. This forces the core to work harder to lift the chest. There'll be an urge to bring the knees fully into the chest—resist it!

CAMEL PULSE

AREAS TARGETED: Core, quads, hips and glutes

Stretch your quads, hip flexors and core all at the same time.

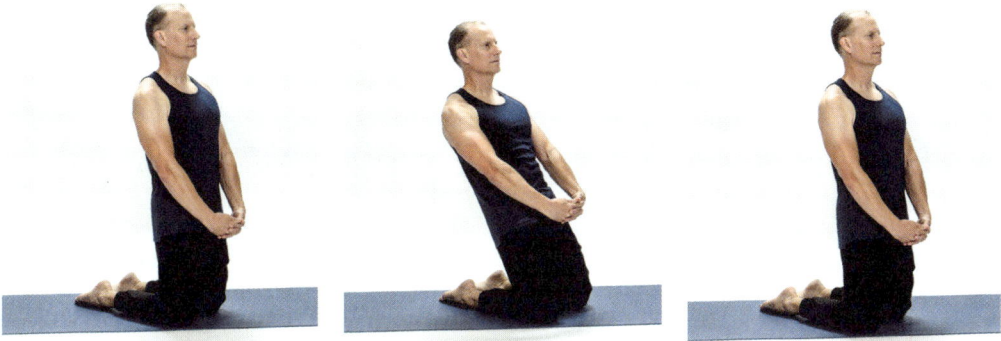

1. Take the same starting position as the Chest Expansion and clasp your hands together in front of you.

2. Draw your chin to your chest and inhale as you hinge back from the knees while staying tall in the spine.

3. Exhale, squeeze your glutes and return to the starting position. Perform 5–10 repetitions.

Key Points

- As in the Chest Expansion, keep a long, straight line from your knees to the crown of your head.

- This is great exercise for your buttocks to shine! Engage and squeeze them throughout the movement.

- The more you lean back, the more intensity you add to this exercise. You will feel a deep stretch in your quads and hips.

PULLING THE T-STRAPS

AREAS TARGETED: Core, back, shoulders and glutes

Turn your attention to building a long, lean strong back.

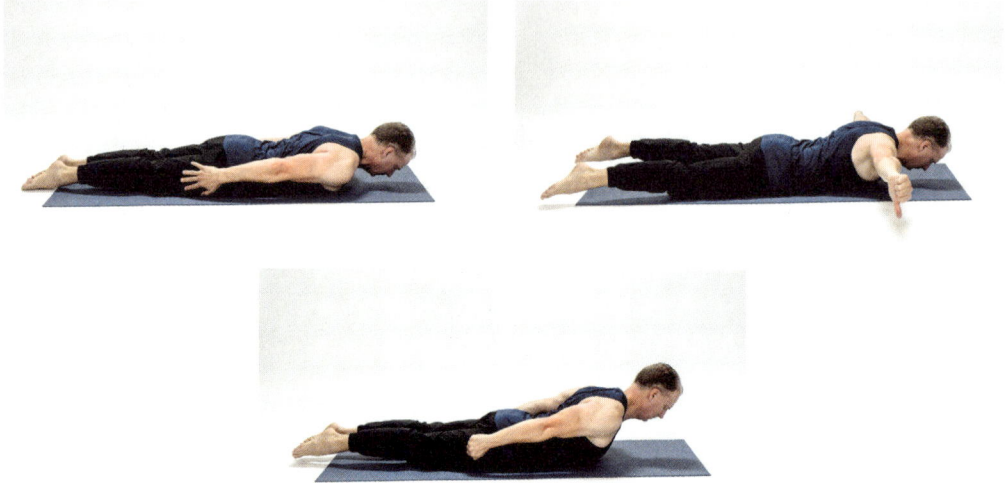

1. Lower down onto your stomach. Bring your arms against your sides and up and squeeze your legs together. Tuck your chin so the back of your neck is long and the crown of your head is extended forward.

2. Inhale, reach your arms halfway forward into a "T" shape while opening your legs as wide as possible.

3. Exhale and return to the starting position. Repeat 5–10 times.

Key Points

- Think of creating long, lean back muscles throughout this exercise.
- Perform the exercise with your hands clenched into fists.
- Lift as much of your upper body off the floor as you can on the exhale.

ONE LEG CIRCLES

AREAS TARGETED: Core, hamstrings and hips.

Improves core stability, hip mobility, and pelvic control while strengthening the abdominal and leg muscles. And it's a beautiful challenge!

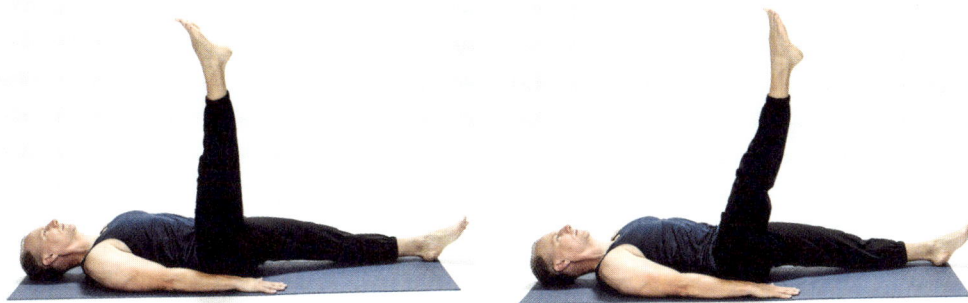

1. Begin lying on your back and arms to your sides on the floor. Extend the right leg to the ceiling and extend the left leg forward onto the ground.

2. Inhale and circle the right leg in a full circle the size of a frisbee to the right and exhale as it returns to the 12:00 position (starting position). Pause for a moment and continue doing 10 circles before reversing the direction for 10 more. Perform on both sides.

Key Points

- Sink both hips down into the mat to avoid needless jostling, which interferes with the flow. Nothing should move except for the leg which is circling. Stabilize the body against that circular movement.

- Sink the shoulders down and away from the ears. Your upper body posture remains solid while sinking the low back into the mat.

- Men may have more of a struggle with this exercise because of a tightness in their hamstrings and low back. Place your hands under your hips, and bend the circling leg or bend the bottom leg with your foot flat on the ground to lower the intensity.

ROWING FROM THE HIPS

AREAS TARGETED: Core, spine, hamstrings, calves, back, arms, shoulders and chest

An obscure exercise which stretches your hamstrings and back and improves posture.

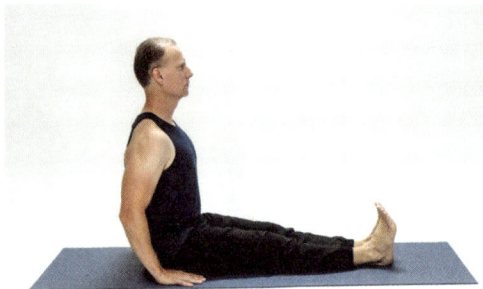

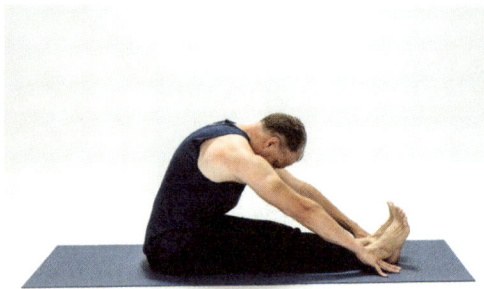

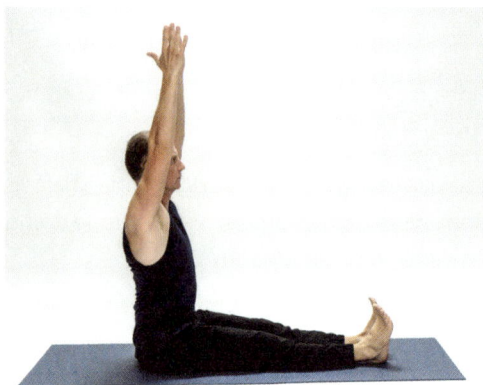

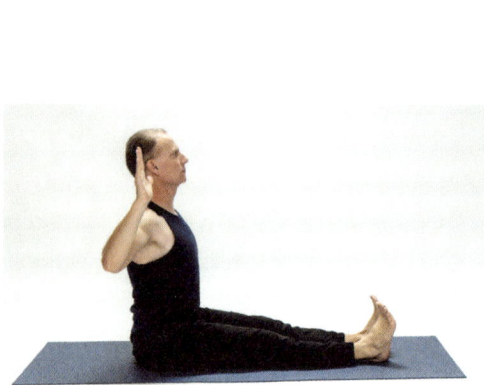

1. Begin in a seated position with your legs extended forward and sitting tall. Release your arms so your fingers brush the ground. Draw your toes towards you and press the backs of your knees down.

2. Inhale prep, exhale and hinge forward while brushing your fingertips on the floor. Tuck your chin and allow the crown of your head to lead.

3. Inhale, activate the abdominals and lift your upper body tall with your arms overhead.

4. Exhale and pull your arms back and down (into what I call "cactus arms").

5. Return to the starting position with an inhale prep. Repeat 5–10 times.

Key Points

- When hinging forward, pull your belly button up and into the spine. Your glutes need to stay on the mat.

- Practice extending further forward with each repetition.

- When doing cactus arms, imagine someone gently pulling your elbows and shoulders behind you. You may hold this position for an extra breath to continue opening the chest, shoulders and breath.

■ PILATES PUSH-UPS

AREAS TARGETED: Core, hamstrings, back, spine, shoulders, chest and triceps

My go-to full body exercise to stretch and strengthen my whole body. Packs a real punch!

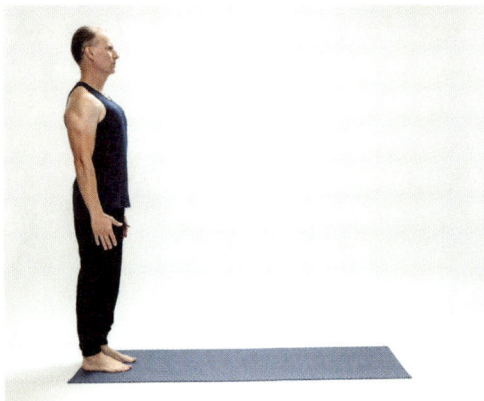

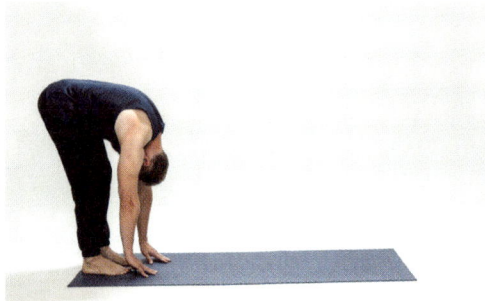

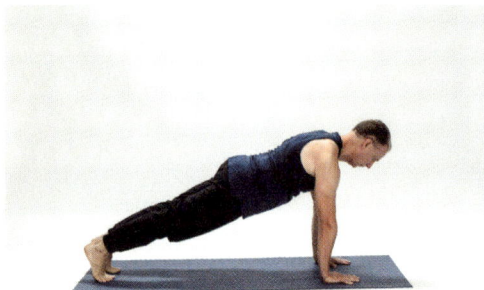

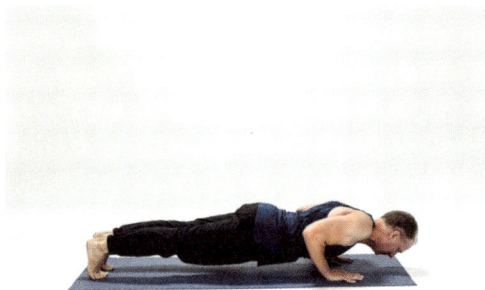

1. Stand on the back part of your mat with your arms to the sides and feet hip-width apart.

2. Inhale and lift your arms overhead into a back bend.

3. Exhale, tuck your chin and dive downward into a forward fold. Lead with the crown of your head and allow your spine to decompress.

4. Continue exhaling as you walk your hands out into plank position, with your hands under your shoulders, elbows turned in and shoulders pulled back and away from your ear.

5. Inhale as you lower into a push-up, keeping your body straight and elbows hugging the sides.

6. Exhale and press back to plank.

7. Continue exhaling and walk your hands back to forward fold while lifting your tail-bone high.

8. Inhale, tuck your chin and roll up to a standing position with a rounded back.

9. Continue inhaling as you lift your arms overhead into a back bend.

10. Exhale, tuck your chin, dive forward and down and continue the exercise. Repeat 5–10 times.

Key Points

- The roll down into forward fold is a golden opportunity to lengthen and strengthen the spine while bringing some fresh, oxygen-filled blood to the brain. Focus on articulating the spine vertebra by vertebra on the roll down and roll up.

- A structured and aligned push-up is parallel to the ground. Add a little extra on your push-up by brushing the chest on the ground on the way down.

- This is a very linear exercise. Keep your movements forward and back, forward and back. Practice so much that this exercise becomes one continuous movement with no beginning and end.

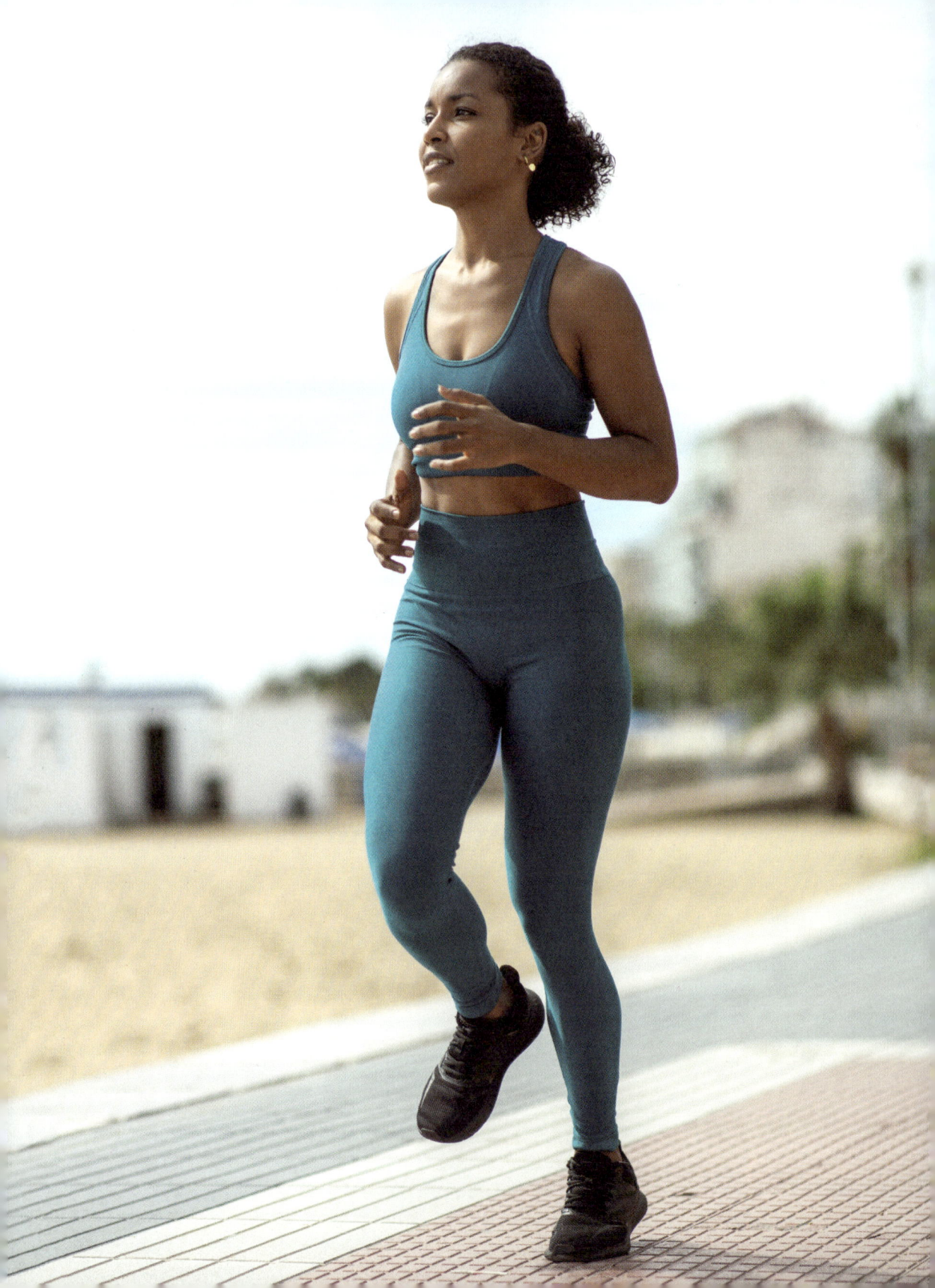

Abdominal Exercises for Runners

Strengthen your core to improve posture,
stability, and stride power on every run.

PILATES 100

AREAS TARGETED: Core, shoulders, adductors and quads

This exercise signals the official start of your Pilates workout—and we're starting with a bang that puts your muscles on notice!

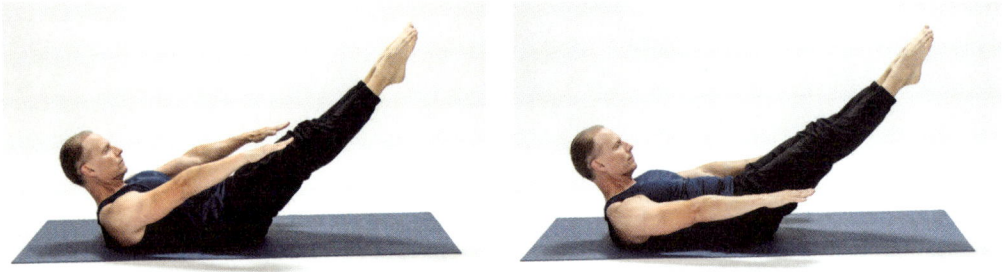

1. Lie on your back, draw your legs to tabletop position and peel the head and shoulder off the mat while raising your arms to the sides. Make sure your low back is imprinted against the mat.

2. Extend the legs and zip them up into Pilates stance with the heels together and feet pointed. Deepen the pull of your abdominals to prepare for the incoming movement.

3. While breathing in for 5 counts and out for 5, pump the arms up and down together about 4–6 inches while sinking the shoulders down and back and expanding the chest. Keep the abdominals pulling into the spine on the exhales. The pumping of the arms is in unison with your breath and will last for 100 counts—hence the name of the exercise.

Key Points

- The Pilates 100 is a beautiful demonstration of core stability in action. The core must work extra hard to stabilize the body against the vigorous movement of the arms. Focus on using your center as an anchor against those pumping arms. You can increase the difficulty by lowering your legs closer to the floor, making your core work harder.

- Keep the chin tucked down towards the chest with enough space in between for a small apple. You will feel a nice stretch in the back of your neck and avoid any undue strain. You may also keep your head on the floor (or use a pillow or rolled up towel) if the strain of lifting your head off the floor is too much. (This applies to all the exercises in this book.)

- All the pumping married with the staccato breaths saturates your muscles with oxygen and strengthens the lungs.

■ SCISSORS

AREAS TARGETED: Hamstrings, core and shoulders

Testing the limits of core and hamstring flexibility.

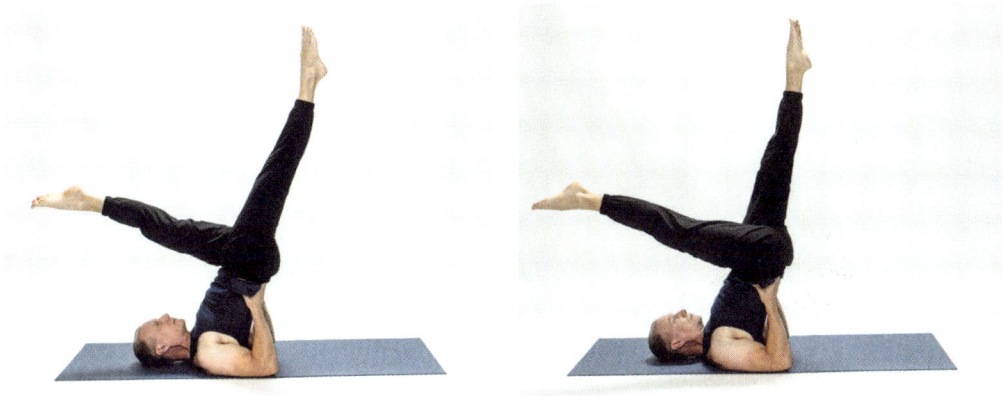

1. Flip over and lie on your back with your legs extended tall to the ceiling and arms at your sides.

2. Activate the abdominals and lift your glutes off the mat while placing your hands on your low back for support. Separate your legs into wide and long scissors. Relax the neck and focus your gaze at the ceiling. Your facial tension must be non-existent.

3. Inhale, scissors the legs and exhale as you scissors again. Repeat 10–20 times total.

Key Points

- If you're a first timer, slow down the movement to avoid tipping and falling on your butt. The combo of the glutes and low back lifting off the floor and legs wildly scissoring back and forth can throw off your balance quickly.

- Don't move your head or neck during the exercise to avoid strain and injury.

- Those of you who practice yoga will recognize the position of the body is similar to shoulder stand pose. There's a little more of a tilt to this one as the shoulder stand is lifted straight to the ceiling.

ROLL UP

AREAS TARGETED: Core, spine and legs

This exercise forces you to get to know your spine and integrate fluidity.

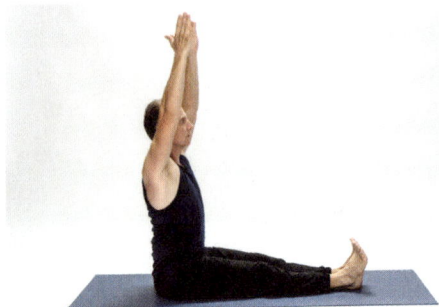

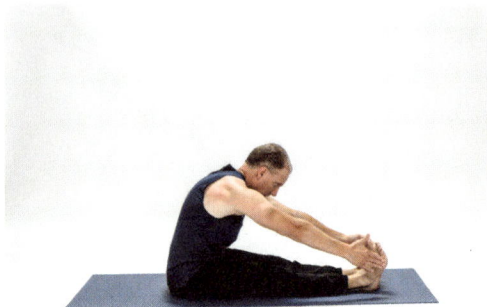

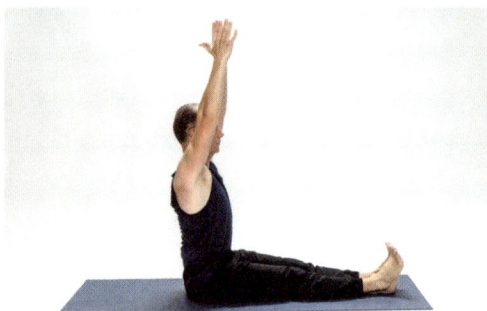

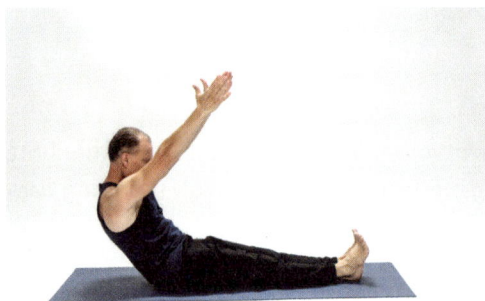

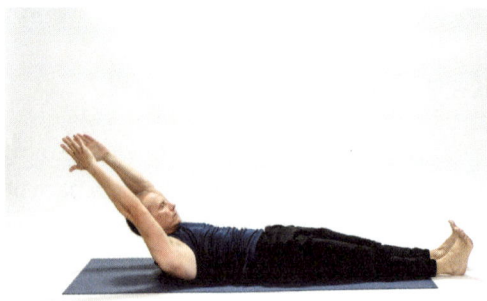

1. Begin seated, with legs extended together. Inhale and reach your arms overhead.

2. Exhale, flex your feet and hinge up and over the legs, bringing your hands to both sides of your heels.

3. Inhale and reverse the exercise as if you're stacking your spine against a wall.

4. Exhale, tuck your chin to your chest and roll down one vertebra at a time, squeezing the legs together.

5. Finish exhaling and extend your arms overhead.

6. Inhale, lift your arms to the ceiling, exhale, and peel your spine off the mat one vertebra at a time. Repeat the exercise 5–10 times.

Key Points

- The roll up needs to be performed at the same speed through the entire exercise. Someone watching you perform it should not be able to perceive where the exercise begins, but rather should see a constant flow. There will be an urge (or necessity) to use momentum at certain points, but practice smoothing those "jerky" movements out. The key word is control.

- Use the "C-Curve" in this exercise, which is the rounding of the back and spine like a wheel (or the letter "C") for the smoothest, healthiest roll down and roll up. You want to fully articulate the spine from top to bottom of the movement. This also means tucking your chin to your chest on the roll up and roll down. This exercise requires a flexible, durable spine.

- Squeeze your legs together for the entire evolution of the exercise to create more stability and add some extra leg work.

- Focus on the contraction of the abdominals to prevent your feet from lifting off the mat. I call it "flying feet." If focus is taken away from the abdominal engagement, the feet will rise and disrupt the flow. Keep your belly button to your spine on the exhales, and keep the foundation in your center.

THE ROLL OVER

AREAS TARGETED: Core, hamstrings, calves and spine

Eliminating the use of momentum is key in this exercise.

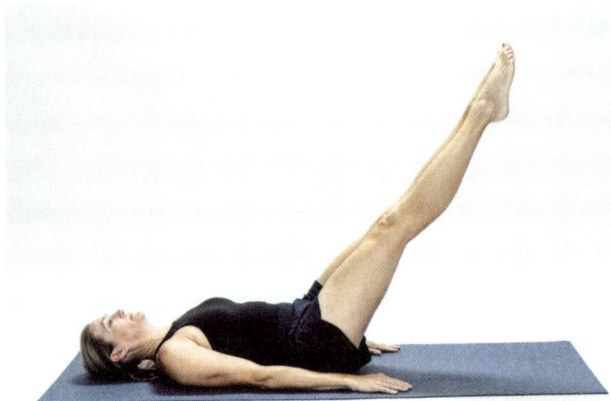

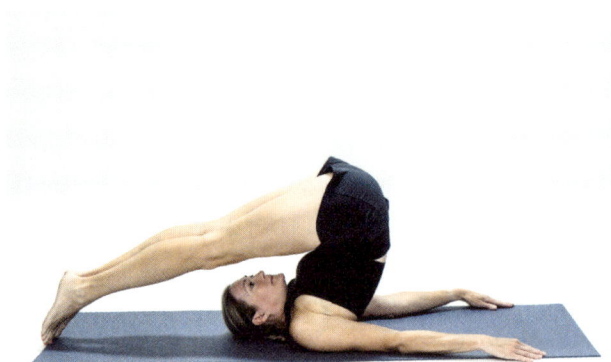

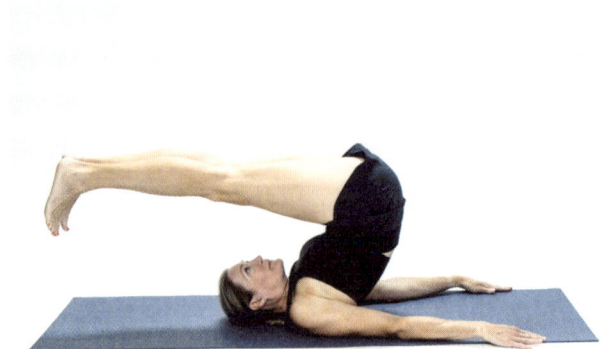

1. Lie on your back, arms against your sides, palms down and legs extended about 45 degrees off the mat. The toes should be pointed, heels together and legs zipped together in Pilates stance.

2. With an electrifying exhale, activate your deep and powerful abdominal muscles to lift your legs up and over your head while smoothly peeling your spine off the mat like a wheel. Touch your toes to the floor.

3. Inhale, lift your toes off the floor and flex your feet, sending a deep stretch down the back of the legs. Continue squeezing the legs together.

4. Exhale, contract the abdominals (belly button to spine) and slowly roll down with extreme control and return to the starting position. Repeat 4–8 times.

Key Points

- Eliminating the use of momentum is key in this exercise. The roll over needs to be fluid and under constant control, which protects the spine from any undue stress and utilizes the core muscles. The arms act as extra support and offer some assistance with the movement, but the emphasis is centered in the powerhouse (core).

- The hips stay evenly aligned and lifted through the movement with the weight of the legs not crushing your chest and stomach. Minimal weight on the head and neck is preferred. Your neck should not feel sore. I teach that the jaw and face are in a neutral, relaxed position. You'd be amazed at how much stress the face can hold and transfer downward through the body.

BACKSTROKE

AREAS TARGETED: Core, hips, inner/outer thighs, arms and shoulders

Another timing challenge to bring the arms and legs together.

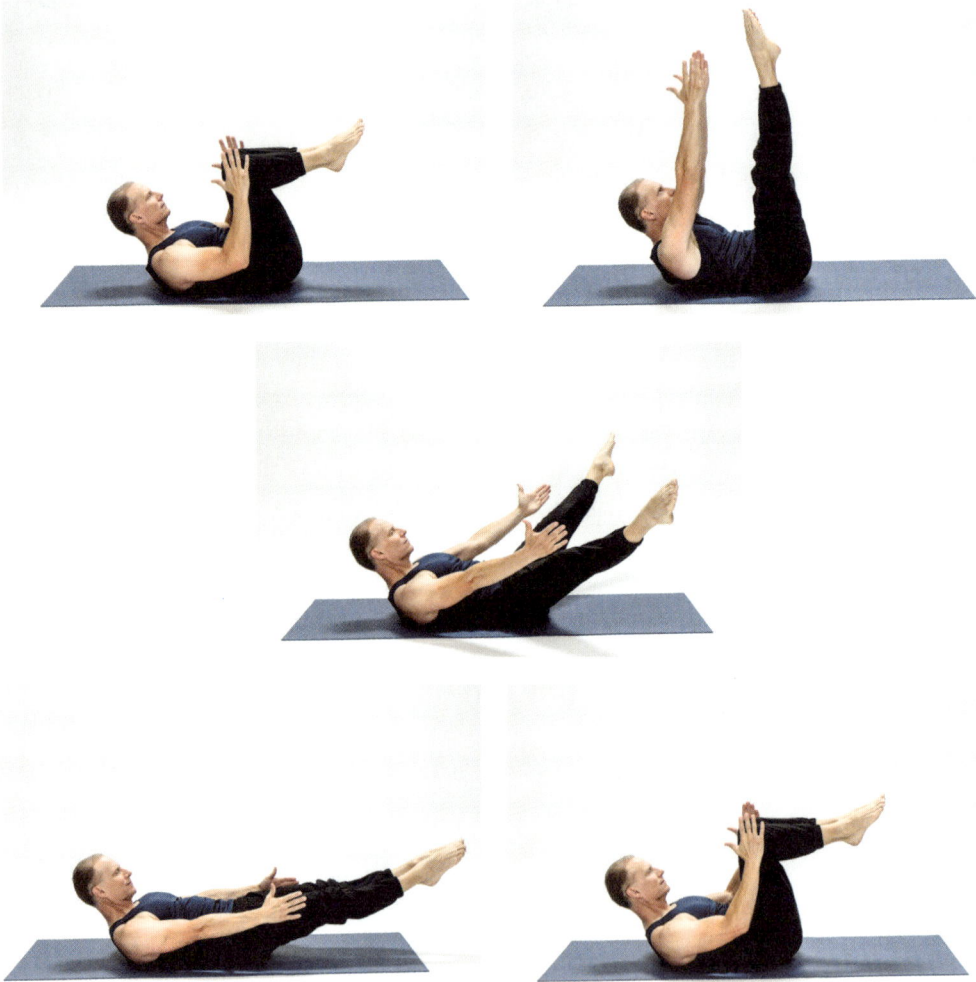

1. Lie on your back with your legs in tabletop position and your arms to your sides, bent at a right angle. Lift your head, neck and shoulders off the mat and tuck the chin.

2. Inhale and extend both the arms and the legs to the ceiling.

3. Continue inhaling as you circle your arms and legs in tandem to the outside.

4. Exhale as you bring your heels together and squeeze your arms against the outside of your legs. Make sure to really give it a good squeeze.

5. Return to the starting position. Repeat 5–10 times.

Key Points

- On the initial upward extension of the arms and legs, reach them to their limit. It's a powerful extra challenge to your leg and low back flexibility and sets the tone for a full and complete circle.

- The lower you bring your legs and arms to the ground, the more of a core challenge you create.

- Work on consistently increasing the size of the circles for more leg and hip flexibility and mobility.

■ CORKSCREW

AREAS TARGETED: Core and legs

An exercise in precision and control.

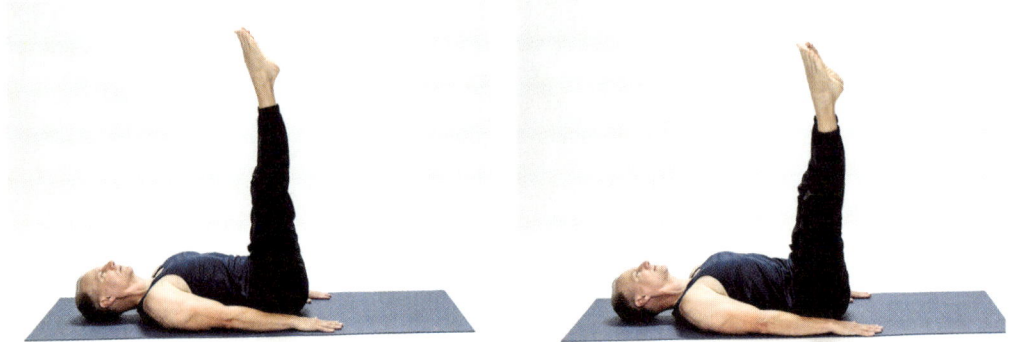

1. Lie on your back and extend your legs to the ceiling. Zip your legs into Pilates stance with heels together and feet pointed. Your head is down and arms on the ground against your sides.

2. Inhale and move your legs to the right in a full circle (the size of a frisbee).

3. Exhale as you return to the starting position (the 12 o'clock position) and pause for a second. Repeat 5–10 repetitions in both directions.

Key Points

- This exercise ripples intensely across the abdominals: rectus abdominis, transversus abdominis and the obliques. Even with a small circle, the intensity can be unbearably challenging. Corkscrew the circles with precision and control.

- Even with the big leg movement happening, the rest of your body is relaxed and aligned. Avoid the shoulders creeping into the ears and stabilize the core.

- Eliminate momentum by slowing it down, especially your toughest spots. Test this by creating larger circles.

STRADDLE CRUNCH

AREAS TARGETED: Core, inner and outer legs, hamstrings and calves

We're working the splits into your athletic training.

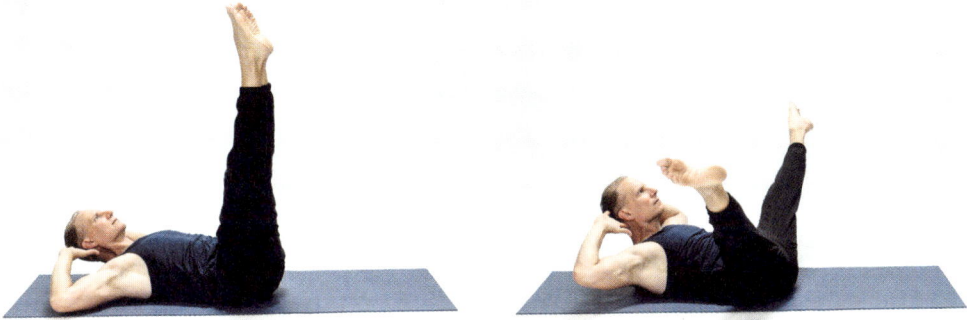

1. Lie on your back with your legs extended to the sky, head, neck and shoulders off the mat and your fingertips gently touching the back of your head. Do not lace your fingers together and let your elbows point outward. Squeeze your legs together.

2. Exhale, lift your chest up into a crunch, point your feet and open your legs as wide as possible.

3. Inhale, flex your feet and return to the starting position. Repeat 5–10 times.

Key Points

- Work on the timing of this exercise. Time it so your chest is lifted and your legs are completely opened at the same time. Also, practice the timing of the return to the starting position.

- Open your legs in a straight line outward and inward with a slight bend in your knees.

- For an extra challenge, you may also extend your arms overhead on the inhale and reach them between your legs on the exhale. Focus on lifting your tailbone off the mat.

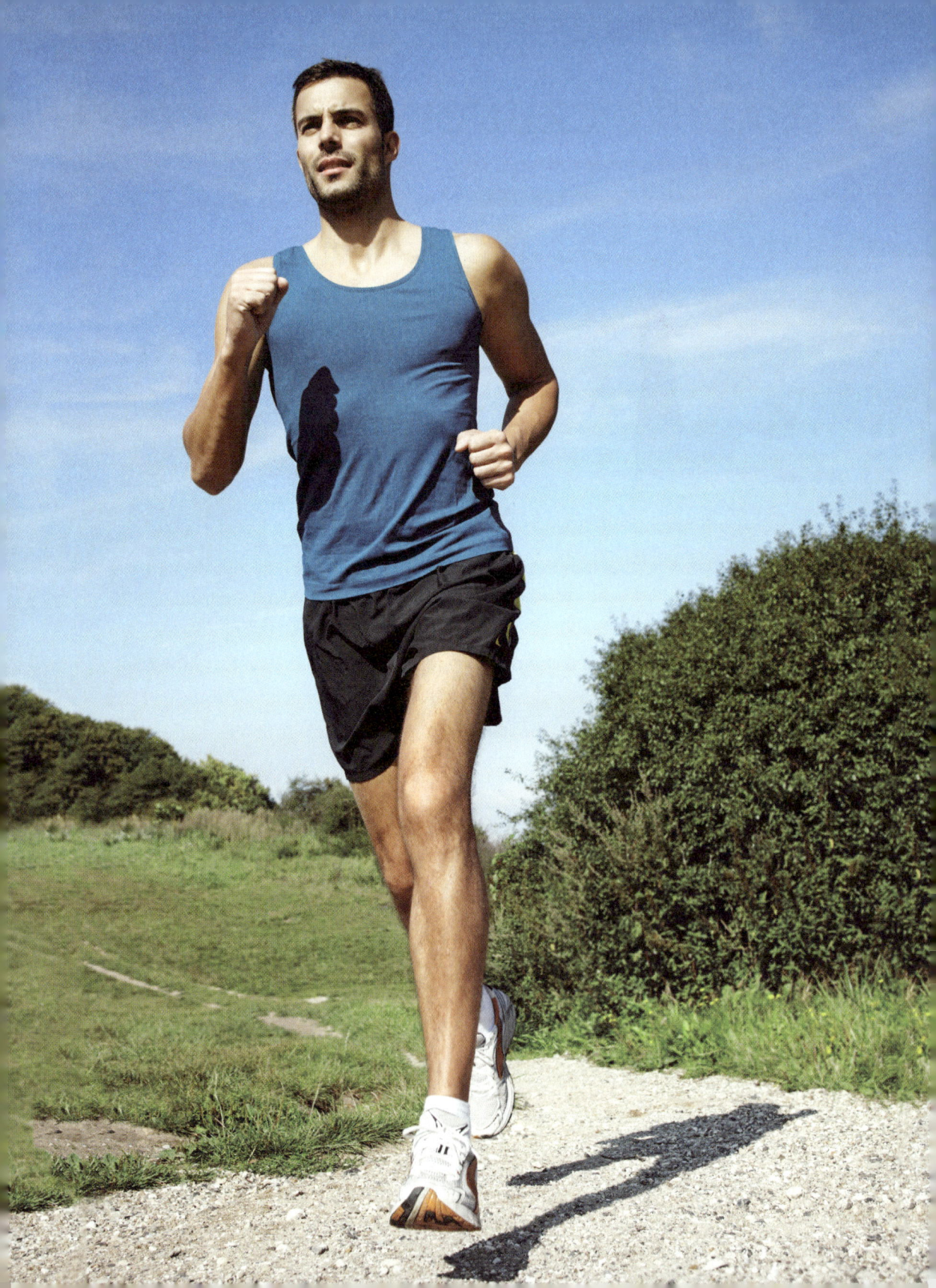

Back & Core Exercises for Runners

Support your spine and reduce fatigue with exercises that target deep postural muscles.

PULLING THE STRAPS

AREAS TARGETED: Core, back, shoulders and glutes

Continue building those long, lean back muscles.

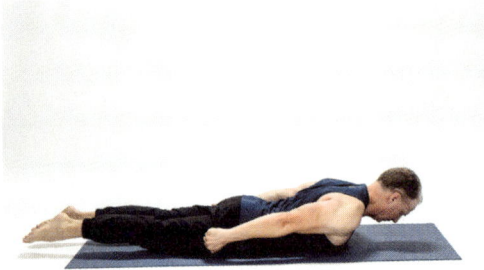

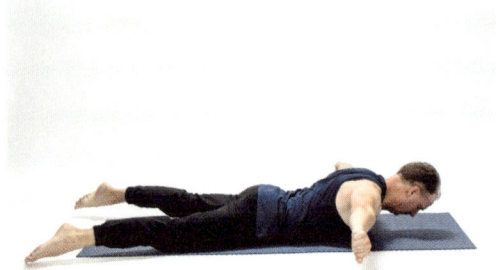

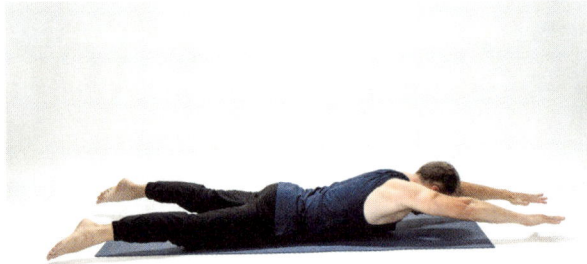

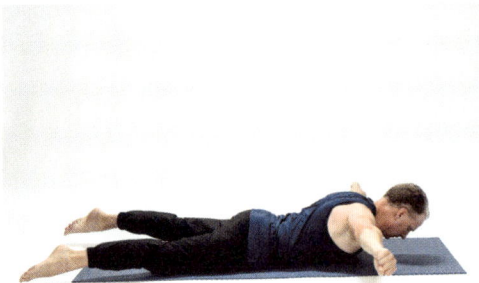

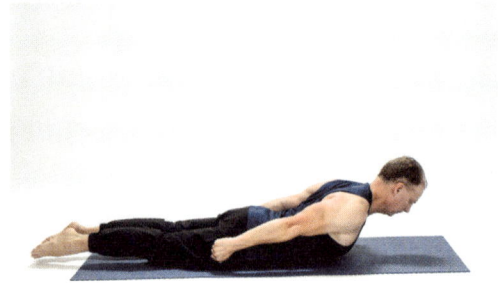

1. Begin on your stomach with your arms to your sides and legs together.

2. Inhale and reach your arms out and all the way forward while opening your legs as much as possible.

3. Exhale and return your arms and legs to the starting position. Repeat 5–10 repetitions.

Key Points

- When pulling your arms to the sides, lift them up as high as you can.
- Squeeze the heck out of your glutes and inner thighs when bringing your legs together.
- Keep your hands in fists throughout the exercise and lift your upper body on the pull back. Add more shoulder mobility each repetition.

SINGLE LEG KICK

AREAS TARGETED: Core, back, hamstrings, quads, calves and arms

Improve upper body posture while stretching the legs. There are no add-ons for this exercise, because why mess with (near) perfection?

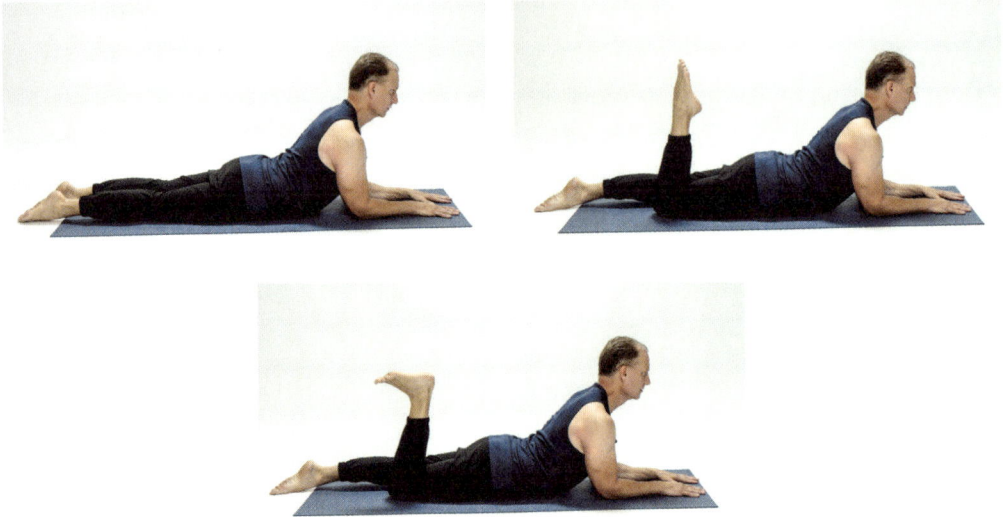

1. Place your elbows under your arms with your forearms pointed forward and hands flat. Extend your legs back with the tops of the feet on the floor.

2. Exhale twice as you kick the right leg from the knee joint twice. Point your foot on the first breath and flex on the second.

3. Deliver your foot to the mat and repeat with the left leg. Maintain a tall chest with your shoulders back and down. Repeat 4–6 times on each side.

Key Points

- Add an extra arm and forearm blast by actively pressing the forearms into the ground.
- Keep abs up and in, even before you begin the kicking. It is easy to disengage the abs in this exercise.
- Keep your eyes focused directly ahead to avoid unnecessary strain on the neck. The jaw is loose.

DOUBLE LEG KICK

AREAS TARGETED: Core, hamstrings, calves, shoulders, quads, back and glutes
We're adding a double kick for a burst of energy.

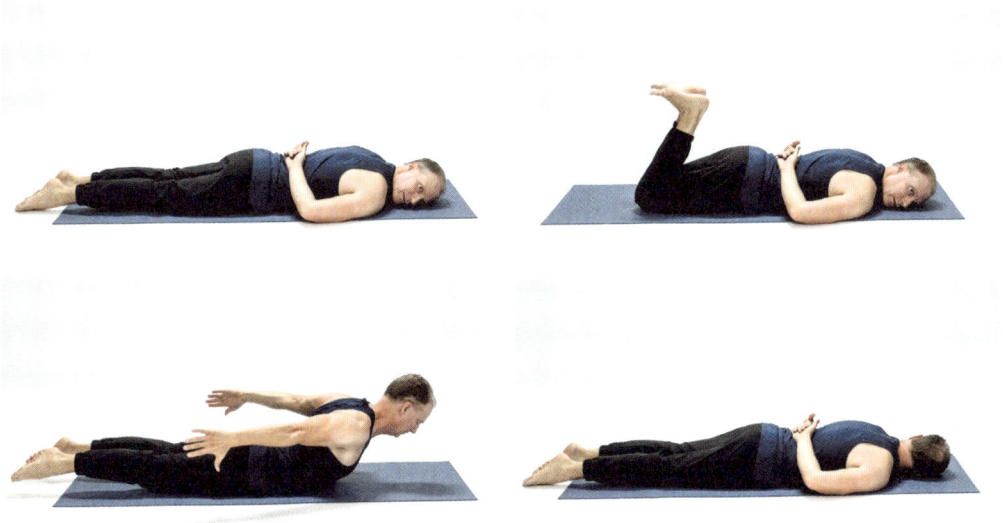

1. Lower onto your stomach, place your hands on your low back and set your right cheek on the floor. Keep your elbows wide.

2. Kick both legs twice (point/flex) with two exhales.

3. Inhale and lift your body off the mat while straightening your legs. Extend your arms behind you. Hold for an extra breath.

4. Return to the floor with your left cheek on the ground and repeat. Do 4–8 repetitions.

Key Points

- There are a lot of moving parts in this exercise, so I recommend breaking them down before attempting to rush through them.

- Be gentle with your head and neck as you continue to place each cheek on the mat. Use control to avoid undue neck stress…or giving yourself a black eye.

- When pumping the legs, you may touch your heels on your glutes, but work your way up to that. Allow the legs and low back to loosen up at their own pace.

SHOULDER BRIDGE

AREAS TARGETED: Core, quads and glutes

To build a sturdy bridge, we need a strong foundation.

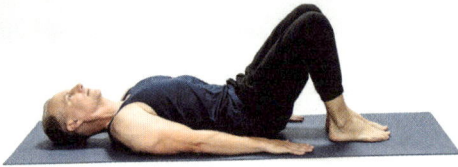

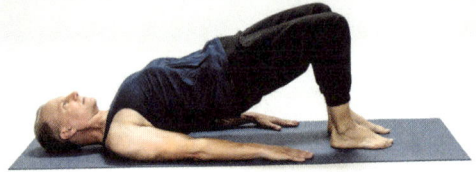

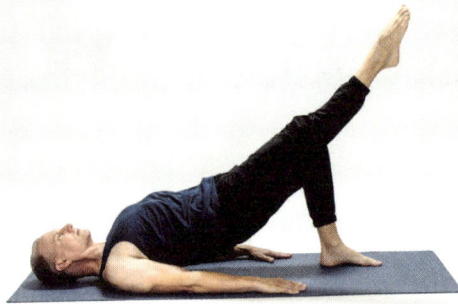

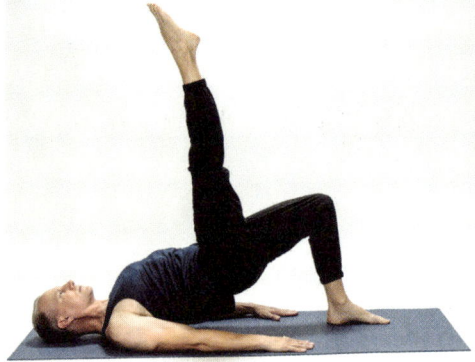

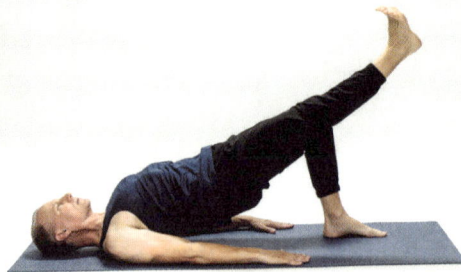

1. Lying on your back, bend your knees and place your feet below the knees. Your feet should be hip-width apart with your arms at your sides against your body.

2. Inhale, tuck your tailbone under your body and lift your spine off the mat one vertebra at a time until the weight has shifted to your shoulders.

3. Extend your right leg so it's in line with the top part of the left and the weight shifts to the left foot. Point that foot.

4. Inhale and lift your right leg to a vertical position.

5. Exhale, flex your foot and pull it back to the original position (Step 3). Repeat 10 times on each side.

Key Points

- Maintain a strong, lifted posture in the bridge through the entire exercise, and maintain a lengthened spine.
- Tuck your chin and relax your neck and face. You should feel a nice stretch down the back of the neck.

DOWN DOG LEG LIFTS

AREAS TARGETED: Core, glutes, shoulders, hamstrings, back and calves

Bringing a touch of yoga with some glute emphasis.

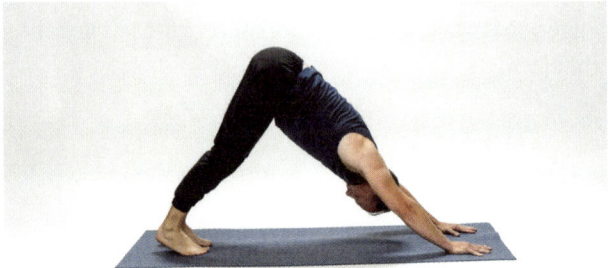

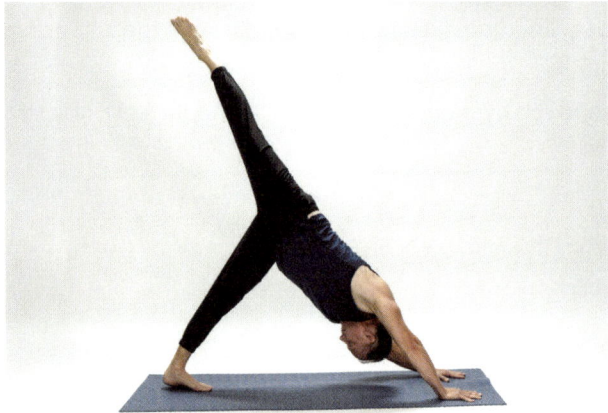

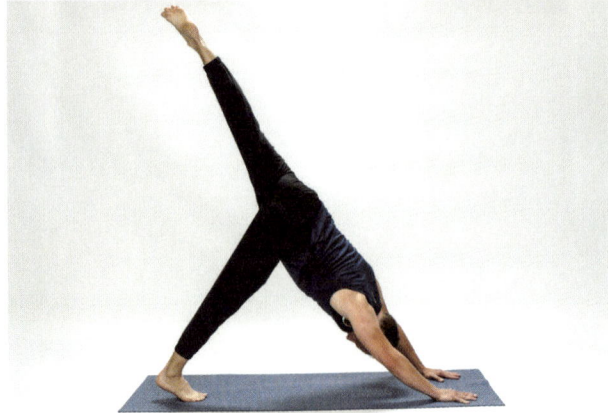

1. Come to Downward Facing Dog with the hands shoulder-width and the feet hip-width apart. Your hands are in front of your shoulders and your feet behind the glutes. Press your upper body towards your legs and sink your heels down towards the ground.

2. Inhale and lift your right leg as high upward as you can. On the top of the lift, open your hip slightly.

3. Exhale and return to downward facing dog.

4. Inhale and lift your left leg to the sky.

5. Exhale and return to downward facing dog. Repeat 10–20 times in total.

Key Points

- I get such a kick out of bringing yoga-inspired variations to Pilates practice. The yoga poses emphasize flexibility, balance and control, and then Pilates comes along and adds an extra core, strength and endurance component. It's a fitness win-win.

- Do not jeopardize your downward dog when you add the leg lifts. If the foundation of the pose breaks down, the whole exercise collapses. Work on a strong foundation first before adding the leg raises.

- Practice moving with the same leg speed up and down without slamming your foot to the ground. I know; we really like to slam those feet down, don't we?

- Spread your fingers wide to draw weight off your wrists and pull your shoulder blades away from each other.

■SWIMMING

AREAS TARGETED: Core, spine, shoulders, glutes and back

Dry endurance swimming at its finest.

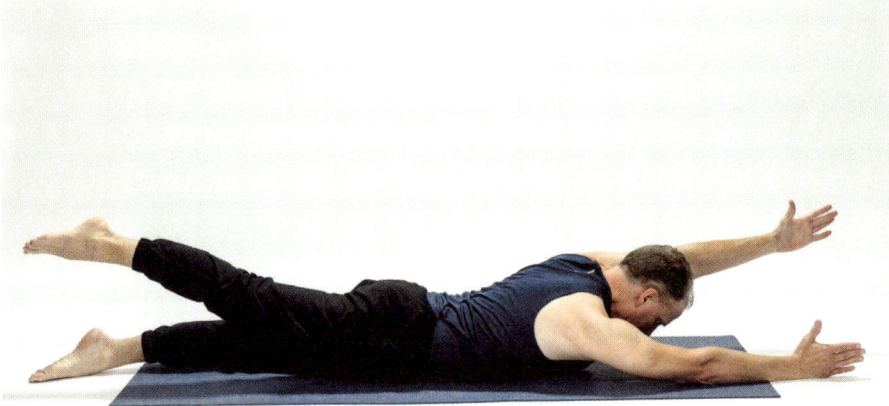

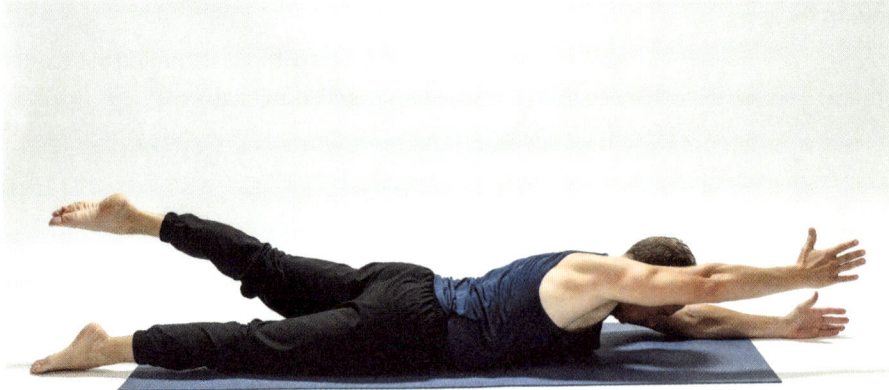

1. Lie down on your stomach with your arms extended long in front, palms facing each other, and legs stretching back. Place your arms shoulder-width and legs hip-width apart. Place your forehead on the mat and point your feet. Lift your hands and feet off the mat.

2. Inhale and lift your right arm and left leg.

3. Exhale and lower them down but not so far as to touch the mat.

4. Inhale and lift your left arm and right leg. Continue alternating the arms and legs for 10–12 repetitions.

Key Points

- Keep your pubic bone pressed into the mat during the exercise and let your eyes focus about one foot in front of the mat.

- Avoid any sort of compression in the spine by continually lengthening into the movement. This includes your low back. Reach your fingers and toes in opposite directions. Allow the crown of your head to stretch forward and lengthen the back of your neck.

- Find the rhythm between the breath and the rising/lowering of your arms and legs.

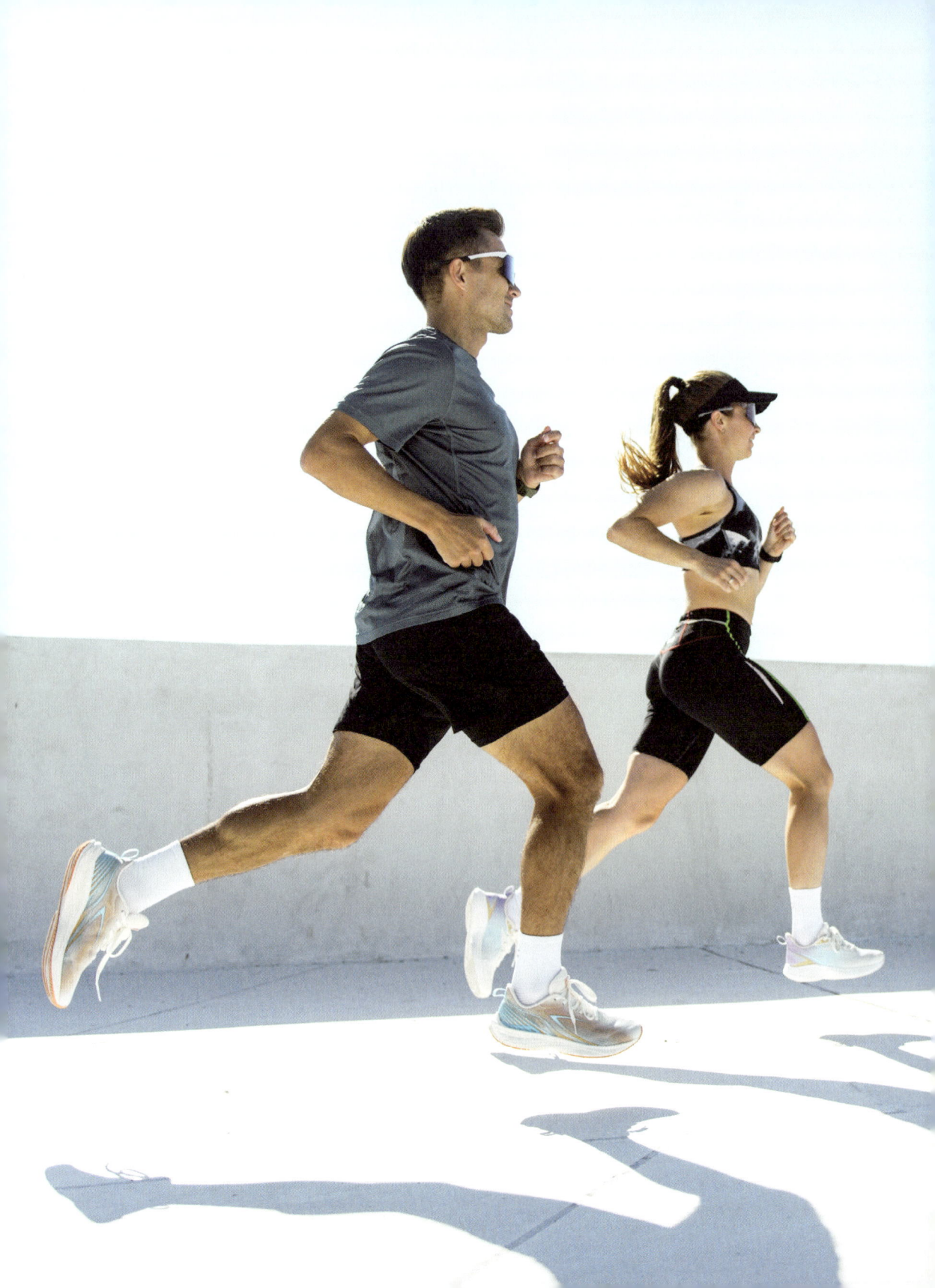

Plank Variations for Runners

Boost total-body strength and endurance with dynamic planks tailored to a runner's needs.

PILATES PLANK

A plank with the Pilates moniker? This must be a power exercise!

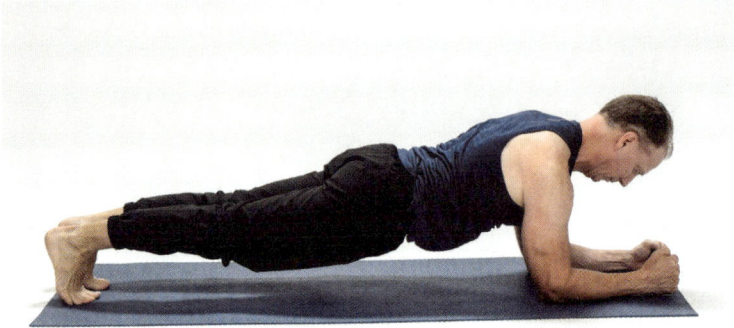

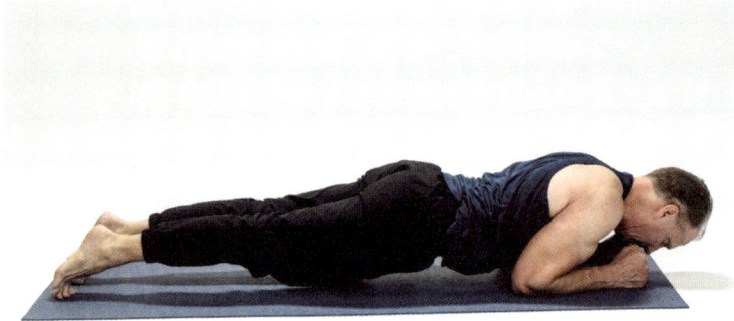

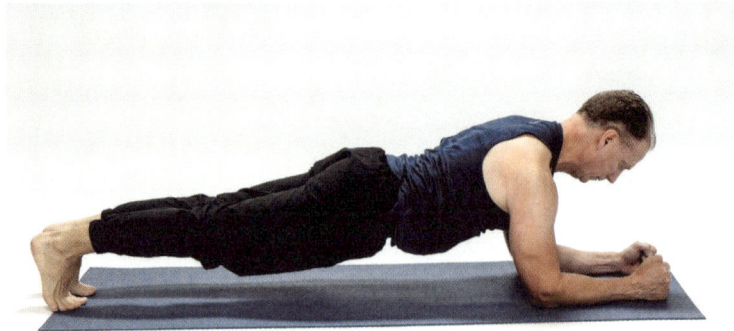

1. Move into a forearm plank with your forearms on the ground, elbows under your shoulders, fingers laced together and heels pressing back behind you.

2. Inhale, press through your toes and shift forward and down, brushing your nose on your thumbs.

3. Exhale and return to the starting position. Repeat for 5–10 repetitions.

Key Points

- As you swoop forward and down for the tender nose brush, give your arms and shoulders a good flex. This is a great way to build extra strength and power.

- You might be tempted to raise your glutes up as you return to plank. Don't—instead, keep a strong plank position throughout the movement to ensure maximum core engagement.

- For a delicious intensity add-on, lift a leg as you move forward and back. Lift the right leg, move forward and down, move back and lower the leg. Alternate with each repetition.

LEG PULL

AREAS TARGETED: Core, glutes, shoulders, triceps and hips

It's called a pull, but we're really kicking it!

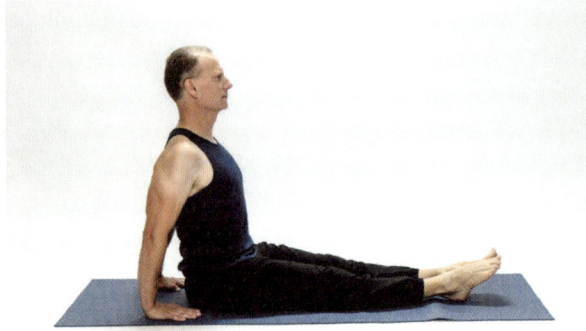

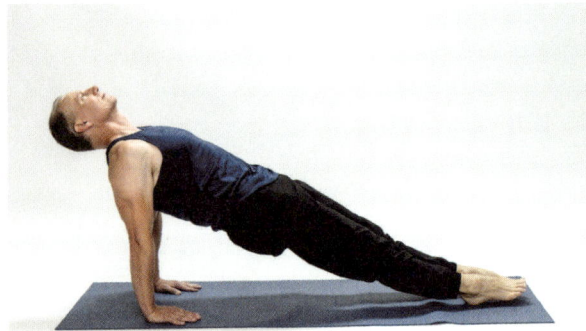

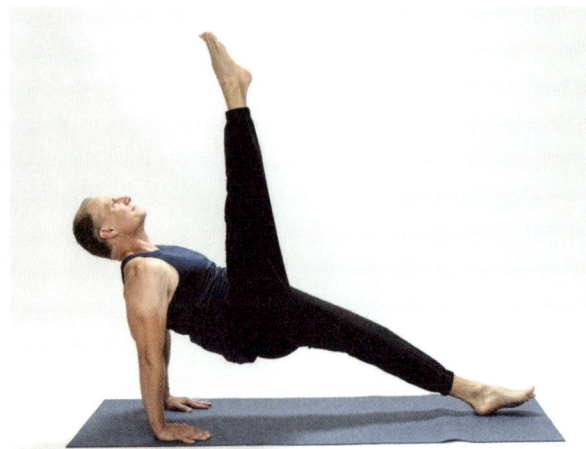

1. Sit upright and tall with your legs extended out in front of you. Bring your heels together and point your feet while zipping up your legs in Pilates stance. Place your hands under your shoulders with the hands positioned in your favored position (I prefer to point the fingers outward but I used to be a fingers pointed towards my butt kind of guy).

2. Press into your hands and lift your hips until your body is in a long diagonal line from your shoulders to the heels. Draw your shoulders back and down and expand the chest. Activate your glutes.

3. Inhale as you kick the right leg up, keeping your body stable and not letting your glutes drop.

4. Exhale, lower the right leg with control, and inhale while kicking the left leg as high as possible. Repeat 6–10 times in total.

Key Points

- The goal with the legs is to kick and raise them higher and higher each repetition while pressing your hands into the ground.

- Your hips and pelvis remain square during the exercise and continue to lengthen the spine and back.

- Beware of collapsing into your chest and shoulders. Focus on opening them to the ceiling to maintain strong posture and open breath.

LEG PULL FRONT

AREAS TARGETED: Core, glutes, shoulders and arms

Give your bum a kicking while stabilizing the rest of your body.

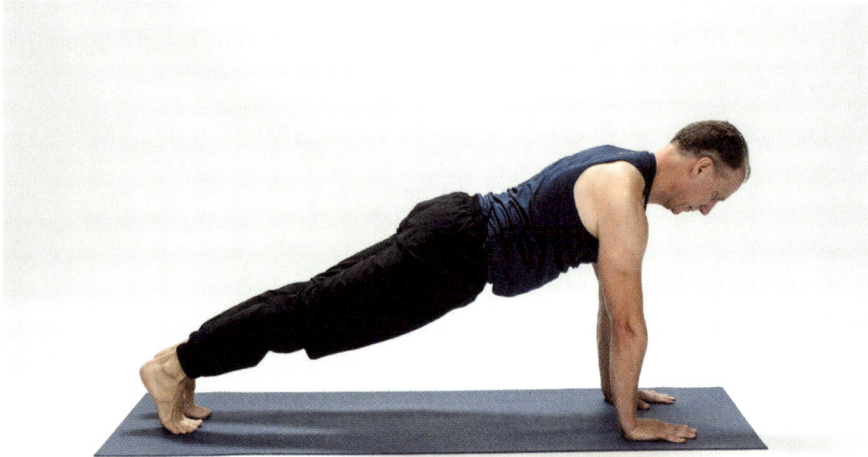

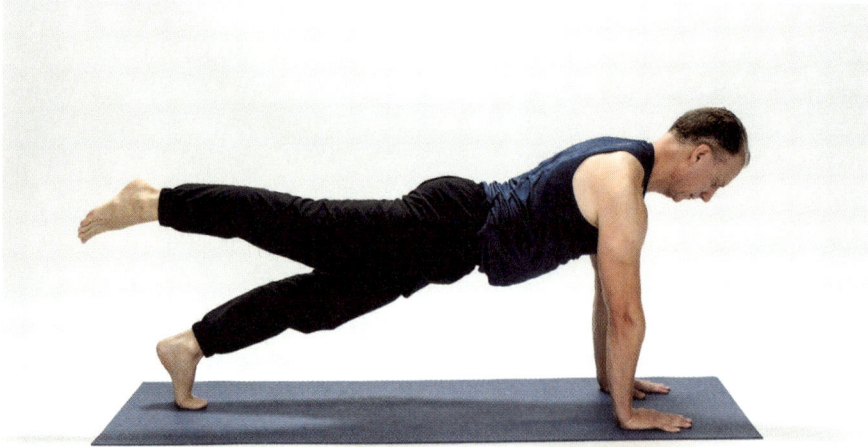

1. Assume a plank position with your hands under your shoulders, shoulders drawn back and chin tucked. Press your heels back for a leg stretch and pull your navel into your spine.

2. Inhale as you lift your right leg.

3. Exhale as you lower the right leg down. Repeat 10–20 times for each leg.

Key Points

- Do not allow your pelvis or stomach to dip during the exercise.

- Your legs need to be the only part of your body which moves. Avoid lifting your pelvis, glutes and low back up and down with your legs.

- Maintain a long, decompressed spine and back during the exercise.

■ STAR

AREAS TARGETED: Core, shoulders and glutes

An advanced plank variation.

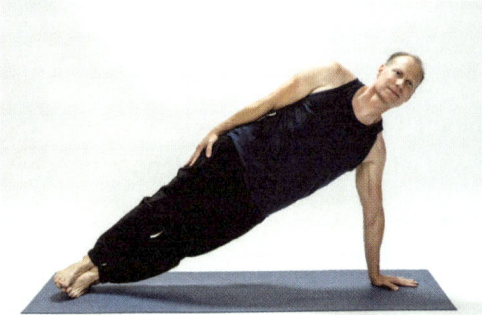

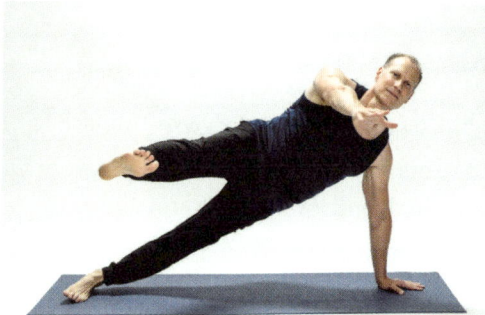

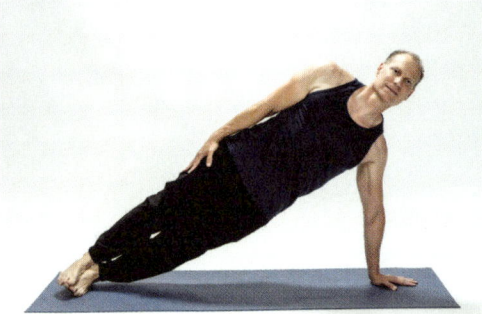

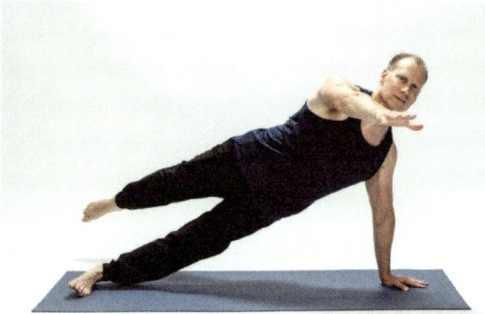

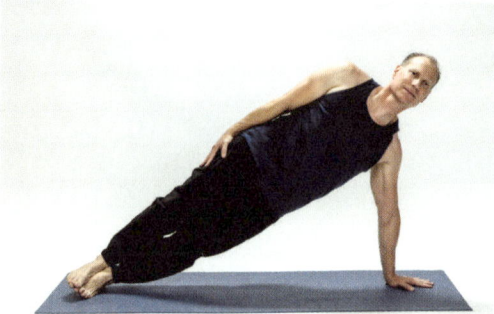

1. Begin in a side plank position, placing your right arm to your side and stack your legs.

2. Inhale and reach your right arm and right leg forward in tandem.

3. Exhale and return to a side plank.

4. Inhale, reach your right arm forward and extend your right leg back. This one takes timing and coordination. Repeat the sequence 5–10 times on each side.

Key Points

- Keep a little softness in the standing elbow to avoid undue pressure on the joint.

- As you move your arms and legs forward and back, maintain square hips and straight legs.

- If you're moving your arms and legs so much that it's destabilizing your side plank, decrease the range of motion. Better to have good, clean form than to attempt more range of motion. "Range is for the ego; control is for the soul."

ELEPHANT PLANK

AREAS TARGETED: Core, hamstrings, glutes, shoulders, chest, calves and triceps

Expand your planks while stretching your legs.

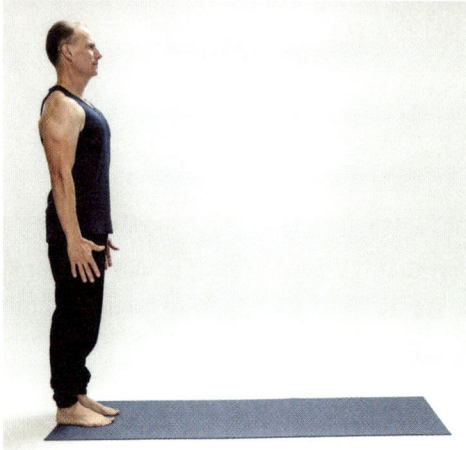

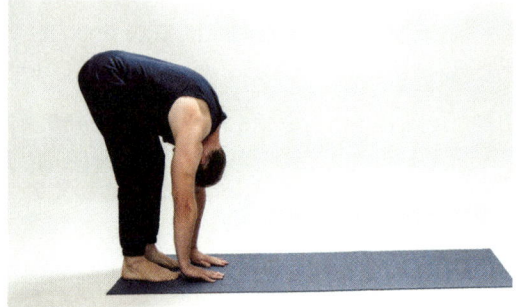

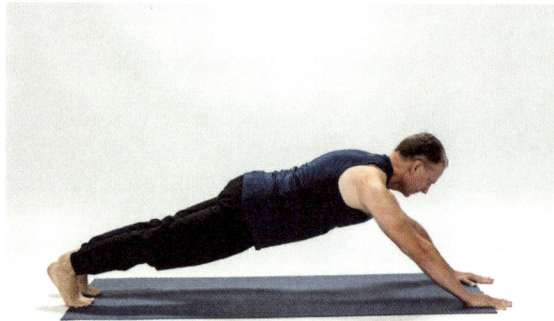

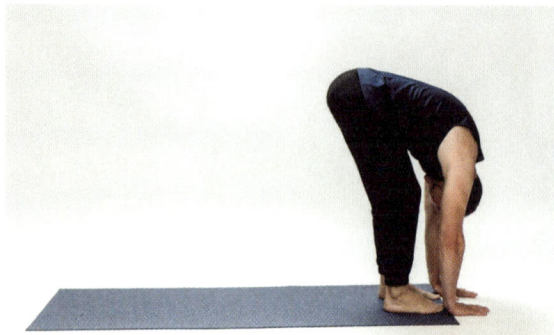

1. From a standing position, exhale and dive forward and down into forward fold. Tuck your chin and allow the crown of your head to sink towards the ground, leaving your arms hanging.

2. Exhale as you walk your hands forward as far as they will go while still maintaining the plank. Hold for a breath.

3. Exhale as you walk your feet forward keeping your legs as straight as possible and pulling the ribs up. Come to forward fold.

4. Inhale, round the spine and rise up to standing position.

5. Exhale and dive down into forward fold.

6. Inhale while walking your feet back to plank. Stretch out the plank as much as possible.

7. Exhale and walk your hands back to forward fold.

8. Inhale and round up into your standing position. Repeat 4–6 times.

Key Points

- The Elephant works best (and is most challenging) when you focus on stretching the backs of your legs throughout the entire exercise. This will push your low back to release and encourage the abdominals to support the movement.

- These are walkout planks, meaning you want to bring your hands in front of your shoulders to place more work and expansion into the abdominals.

- Press through your heels when walking for an extra burn to your calves.

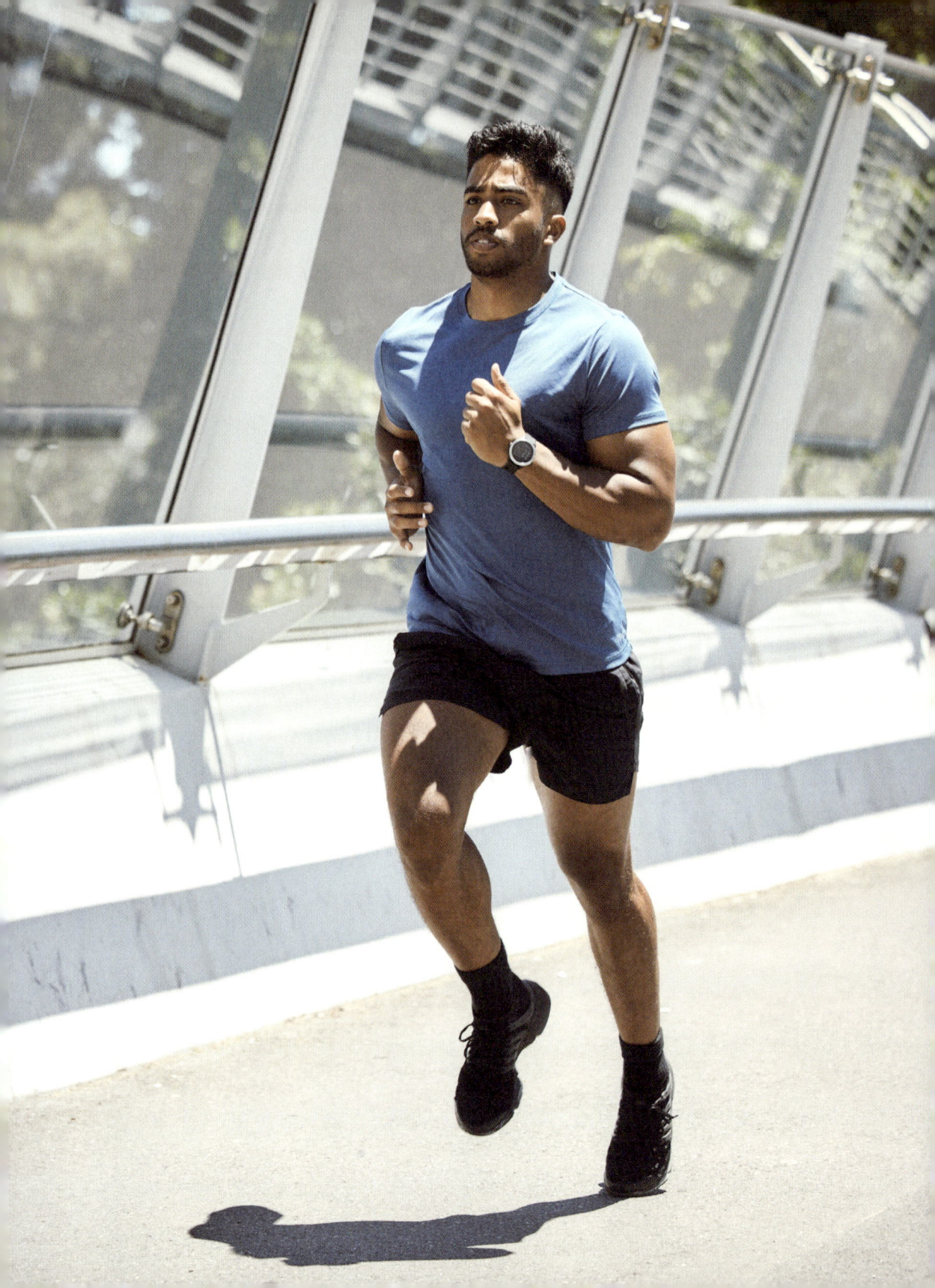

Rowing Series & Seated Core Work for Runners

Enhance breath control, core coordination, and upper-body alignment for smoother runs.

ROWING FROM THE STERNUM

AREAS TARGETED: Core, spine, hamstrings, calves, back, arms, shoulders and chest

How far can you roll back without touching the ground?

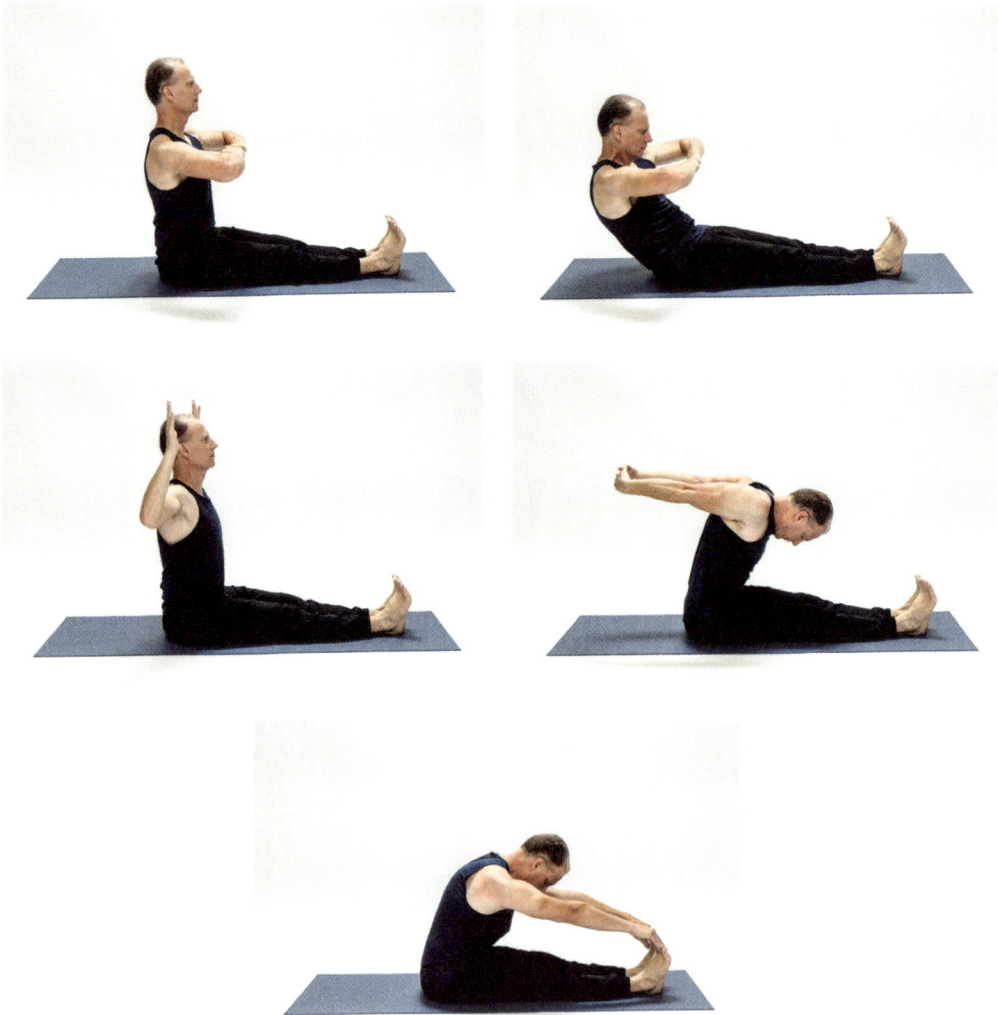

1. Begin in a seated position with your legs extended forward and sitting tall. Make fists and push them together in front of your body at chest level. Point your elbows outward. Draw your toes towards you and press the back of your knees down.

2. Exhale, round your back into a C-Curve, tuck your chin and roll halfway back while squeezing your abdominals. Squeeze your legs together with great vigor.

3. Inhale and sit up tall while reaching your arms up and back.

4. Continue inhaling and lace your fingers together behind as you tuck your chin and lead with the crown of your head.

5. Exhale and extend your arms around and forward with your hands grabbing your toes, feet or ankles.

6. Inhale and return to the starting position. Repeat 4–6 times.

Key Points

- Work on sinking lower in Step 2 with every repetition.
- Flex your arms and shoulders as you roll back and up for an extra muscle toner.
- When switching the arms forward and back, expand your range of motion with progressively larger circles.

ROWING 90 DEGREES

AREAS TARGETED: Core, spine, hamstrings, calves, back, arms, shoulders and chest

Let's get the arms involved.

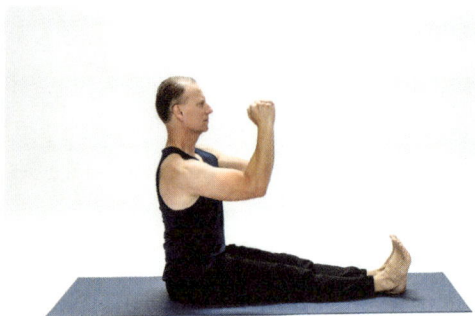

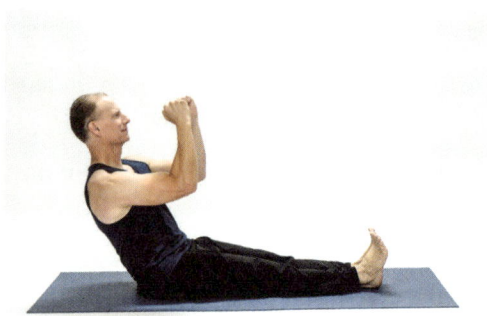

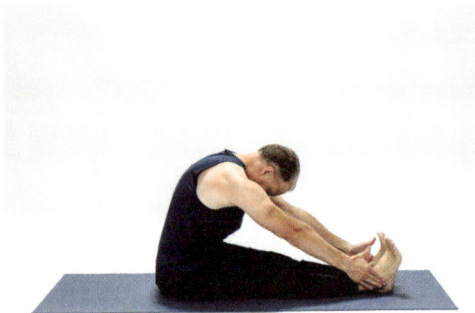

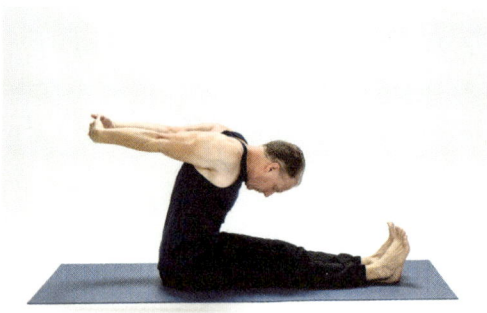

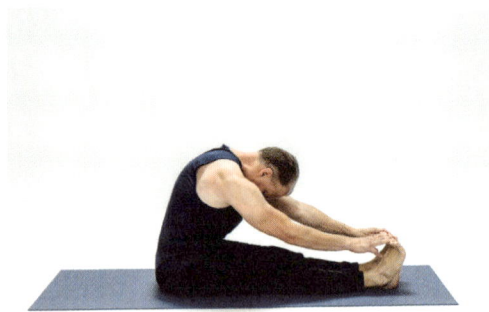

1. Begin in a seated position with your legs extended forward and sitting tall. Lift your arms in front of you and bend them at a 90 degree (right angle) angle with clenched fists, palms facing towards each other. Your arms should be shoulder-width apart. Press the backs of your knees down and draw your toes towards you.

2. Exhale as you hinge back, keeping your spine long with no C-Curve. Go as far as you can without losing your upper body posture.

3. Inhale as you lift tall and extend your arms up and behind you in a circle.

4. Continue inhaling as you hinge your upper body forward and lace your fingers together behind you in a mudra position. Lead with the crown of your head and tuck your chin.

5. Exhale as you reach your arms forward and grab your toes, feet or ankles. Press the backs of your knees down.

6. Inhale and return to the starting position. Do 4–6 repetitions.

Key Points

- Imagine your core is a block of granite on the hinge back—no rounding or C-Curve of the spine allowed. For a tougher core challenge, hold the bottom of this position for an extra breath.

- Flex your arms and shoulders on the roll back for an extra muscle toner.

- When switching the arms forward, up and back, expand your range of motion with progressively larger circles.

◼ SPINE TWIST

AREAS TARGETED: Core and shoulders

We're really wringing out the lungs now.

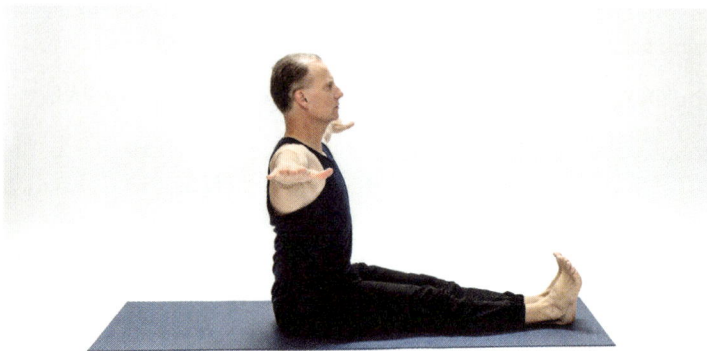

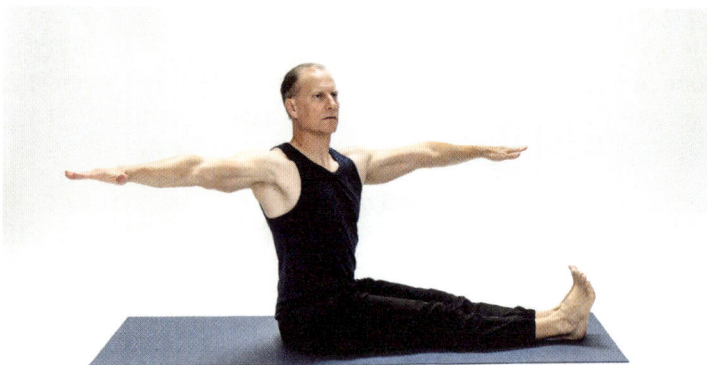

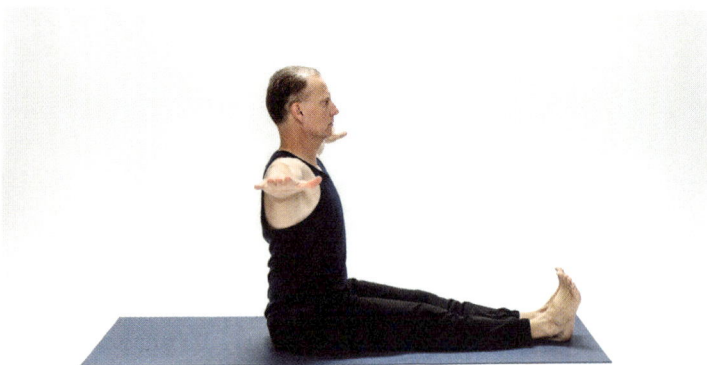

1. Sit up tall and extend your legs straight in front of you. Extend the arms out to your sides in a straight line with your shoulders back and down, chest open and lifting up in the waist. Pull your shoulder blades together in the back. Inhale to prep.

2. Exhale twice as you pulse your upper body to the right 2 times. The first pulse takes you part way into the twist and the second brings you to the farthest possible point of the twist. The second exhale also squeezes every ounce of breath from the lungs. Keep your tall posture.

3. Inhale, return to the center and continue on the other side. Do 5–10 repetitions.

Key Points

- The head and neck stay in line with the spine in this exercise and the crown of the head is lifting upward. The chest is expanded through the exercise.

- Imagine squeezing a dollar bill between the shoulder blades to reinforce a tall, proud posture.

- Minimize the movement of the legs while twisting. This is a full body exercise with all the parts working together in unison.

◾ ROLLING LIKE A BALL

AREAS TARGETED: Core, spine and lungs

We're putting your Pilates "C-Curve" proficiency to the test.

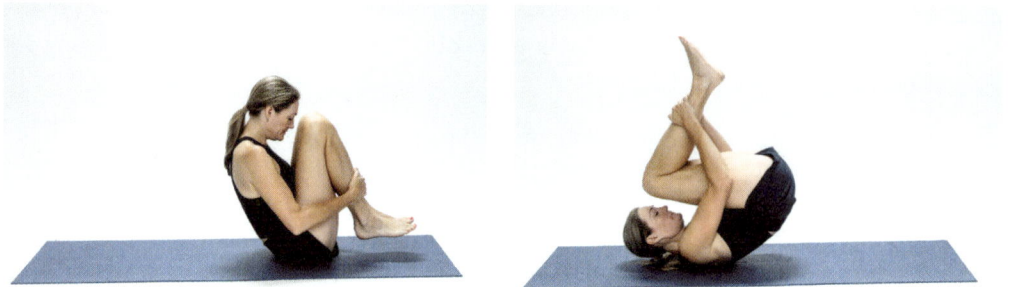

1. Begin in a seated position and draw your knees towards you, lifting your feet off the mat and placing your hands on your ankles or knees. Tuck your chin and round the upper back in a "C-Curve."

2. Inhale and roll back one vertebra at a time until you make contact with your shoulders.

3. Keeping your chin tucked and back rounded, exhale and reverse the roll back to the starting position. Hold and balance that position for a breath before resuming the exercise. Do 4–6 repetitions.

Key Points

- Your goal for this exercise is to do it as slowly and effortlessly as possible.

- In addition to rolling back to the shoulders, your butt and feet need to be pointed towards the ceiling to ensure good posture. Allow your shoulders and arms to be relaxed through the movement.

- Think small. Imagine your body is a very small ball rolling up and down. This visual will help with the flow. Keep your head close to your knees and stay in a straight line up and down. No momentum, no jerky motions; smooth and fluid is healthy for the spine.

BOAT TWISTS

AREAS TARGETED: Core and shoulders

Anytime we add Boat, you know you're going to have to work overtime to maintain the pose, breath and balance.

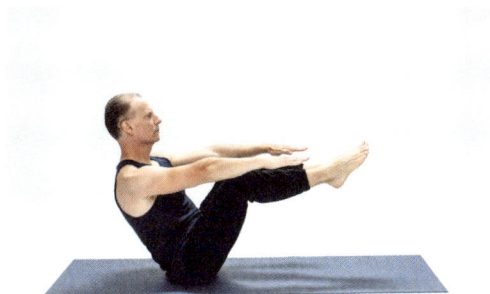

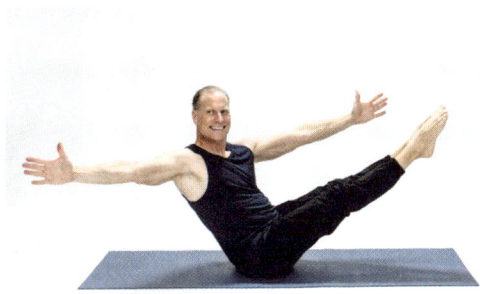

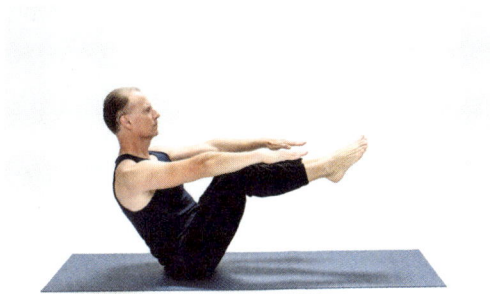

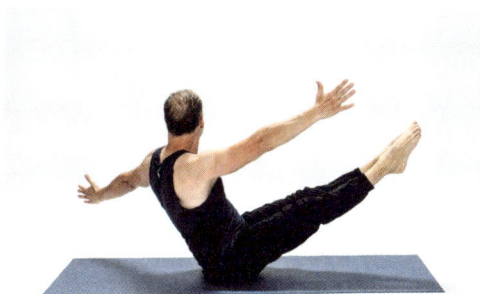

1. Move into Boat position with hands reaching forward and legs at a right angle.

2. Exhale, extend your legs and twist your upper body to the right while opening your arms.

3. Inhale back to Boat position.

4. Exhale and twist to the left. Repeat 6–10 times in total.

Key Points

- There's lots of balance in this twist, so move slowly and hold it for an extra breath. You're balancing on your glutes.

- Squeeze your legs together on the extension and pinch your shoulder blades together on the twist.

- Return to a proper Boat position with your legs at a right angle, arms to the sides and your upper body sitting tall.

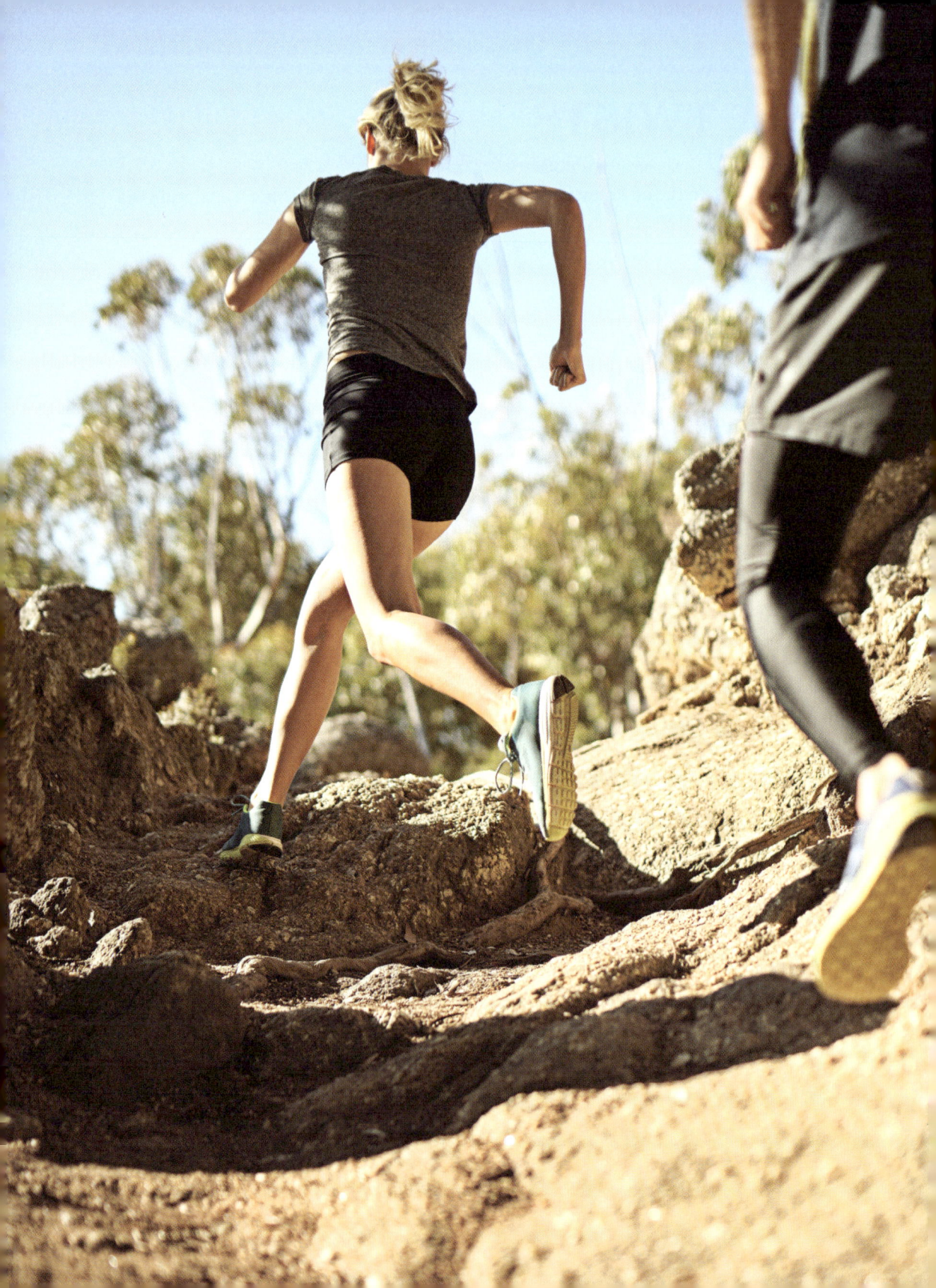

Hip & Leg Exercises for Runners

Activate and balance your hip stabilizers to prevent common running injuries and improve stride efficiency.

CIRCLES

AREAS TARGETED: Core, hips, glutes and hamstrings

These are very deceptive, so proceed with caution…and copious amounts of breath.

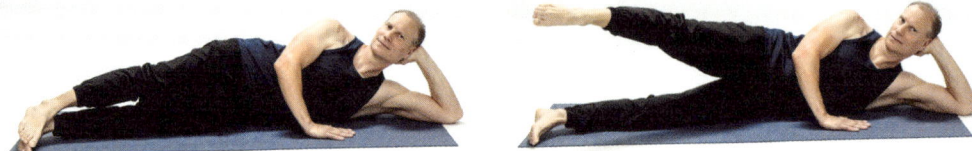

1. Lie on your left side and line up a straight line from the ears to the ankles. Bring your legs slightly forward and stacked to help with balance. Place your left arm on the floor and bend your elbow so you can place your head in your hand. The right hand is placed on the mat for a little extra balance or on your right hip for less.

2. Lift your right leg parallel with the ground. Circle it forward 10 times, drawing a circle the size of a frisbee. You may also tighten up the circle into a tiny one or hit the boundaries and go for a very wide one. Whatever the size, draw with control and precision. Circle the leg 10 times in the other direction.

TAPS

AREAS TARGETED: Core, hips, glutes and hamstrings

Yes, Pilates has exercises for your legs—lots of them!

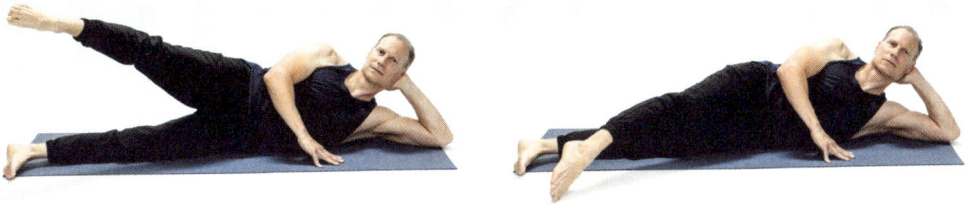

1. Lie on your left side and line up a straight line from the ears to the ankles. Bring your legs slightly forward and stacked to help with balance. Place your left arm on the floor and bend your elbow so you can place your head in your hand. The right hand is placed on the mat for a little extra balance or on your right hip for less.

2. Inhale and lift your right leg parallel with the ground. Exhale and tap your toes in front of you.

3. Inhale and swing your leg behind you and give a light tap. Swoop the leg high in the center and bring it down with beautiful control on the taps. Do 10–20 repetitions in total.

■ KICKS

AREAS TARGETED: Core, hips, glutes and hamstrings
Maintain a straight line in this movement.

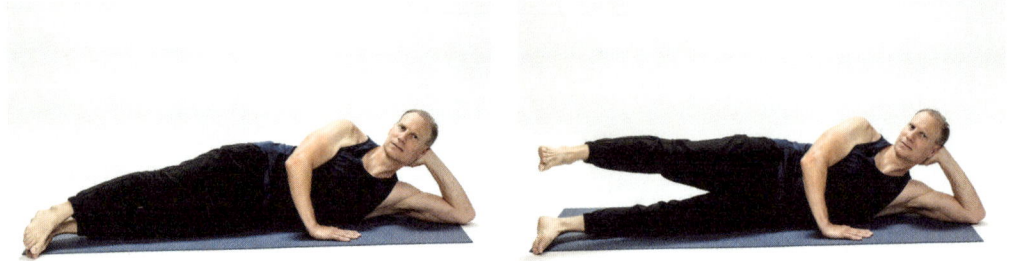

1. Lie on your left side and line up a straight line from the ears to the ankles. Bring your legs slightly forward and stacked to help with balance. Place your left arm on the floor and bend your elbow so you can place your head in your hand. The right hand is placed on the mat for a little extra balance or on your right hip for less.

2. Lift your right leg parallel with the ground. Point your right foot, inhale and kick your leg forward in a straight line.

3. Exhale, flex your foot and pull it back behind you, maintaining the straight line. Do 10–20 repetitions.

KICK UPS

AREAS TARGETED: Core, hips, glutes and hamstrings

It's all about control.

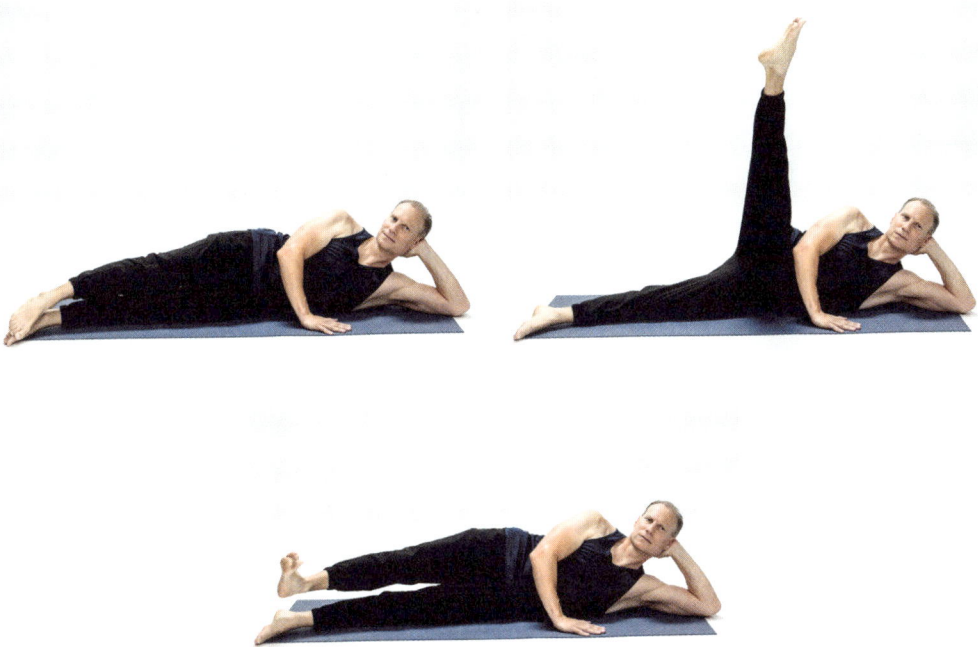

1. Lie on your left side and line up a straight line from the ears to the ankles. Bring your legs slightly forward and stacked to help with balance. Place your left arm on the floor and bend your elbow so you can place your head in your hand. The right hand is placed on the mat for a little extra balance or on your right hip for less.

2. Inhale, point your right foot and kick your right leg to the sky.

3. Exhale, flex your foot and lower your leg with control. Do 6–10 repetitions.

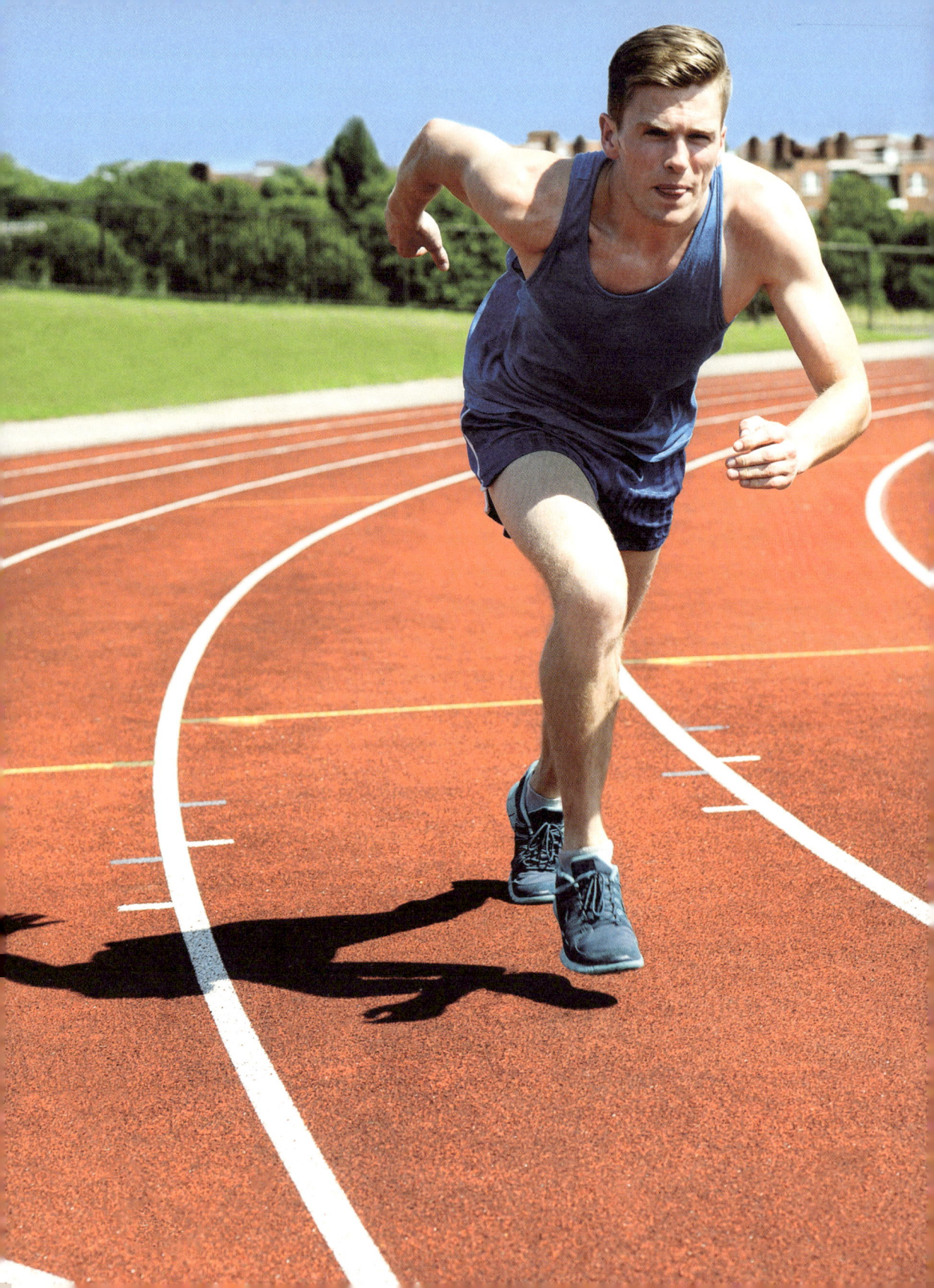

Post-Run Exercises for Runners

Cool down with intention—restore alignment,
release tension, and prepare for your next run.

■ CHEST EXPANSION

AREAS TARGETED: Core, chest, upper back, shoulders and neck

A very effective exercise for increasing breath efficiency and improving posture.

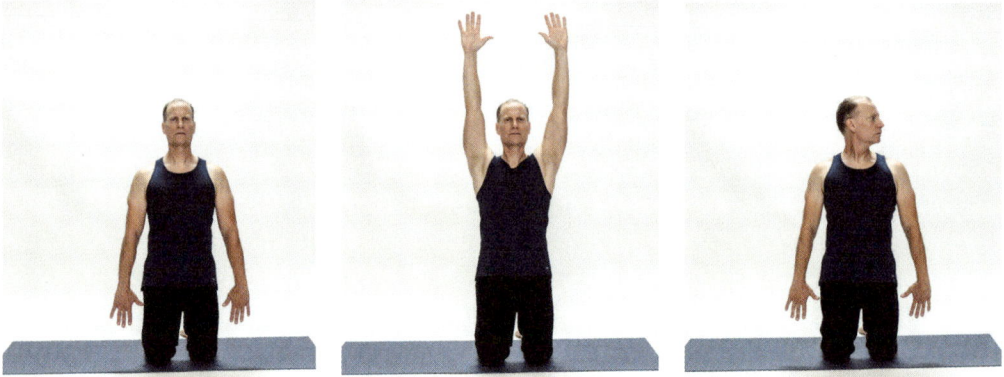

1. Bring your knees hip-width to the mat and place the tops of your feet flat on the ground behind you. Extend your arms down the sides and slightly behind your body with your palms facing back. Sink your shoulders back and down and open the chest. Tuck your chin and lengthen up through the crown of your head.

2. Inhale and lift your arms up and behind you.

3. Exhale and press your arms down and behind you and hold the pose. Turn your head right, left and forward while holding your breath. Inhale, lift your arms up and behind your head and repeat 5–10 times.

Key Points

- Keep your shoulders back and down and spine long through the movement. Pull the abdominals into the spine on the exhale.
- Stay tall from your knees to the crown of your head, even when your arms reach up and behind the body.
- Maintain a long, smooth neck on the head twists.

BIRDDOG

AREAS TARGETED: Core, spine, shoulders, glutes and back

A wonderful exercise to ease you into swimming.

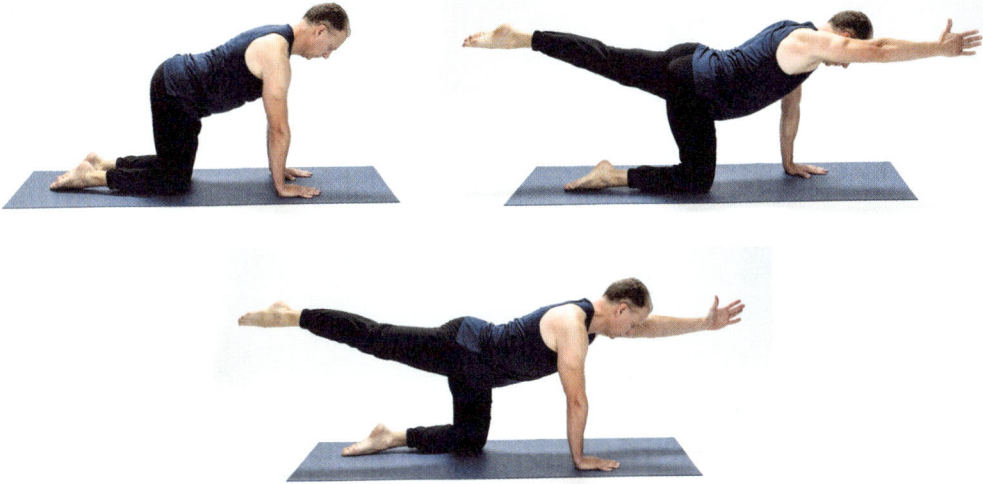

1. From hands and knees position, inhale and extend your right arm and left leg.

2. Exhale as you return them to the mat. Repeat on the other side 10–20 times.

Key Points

- Try to extend your arm and leg in a straight line, extending the fingers and toes away from each other.
- For a greater challenge perform this exercise with your hands on the floor in front of your shoulders. It forces your core to stabilize more against the movement.

SNAKE

AREAS TARGETED: Core, hips and spine

Bringing lots of spinal flexibility with this yoga-inspired Pilates move.

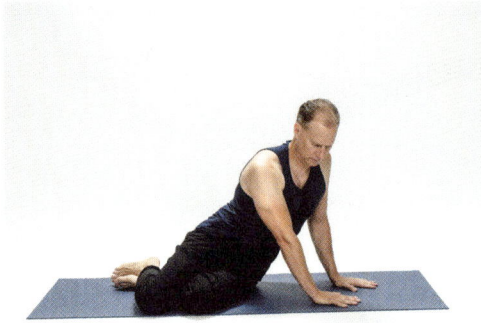

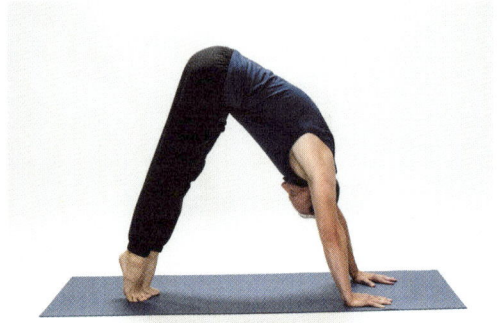

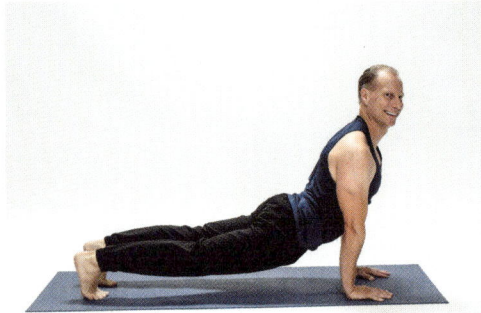

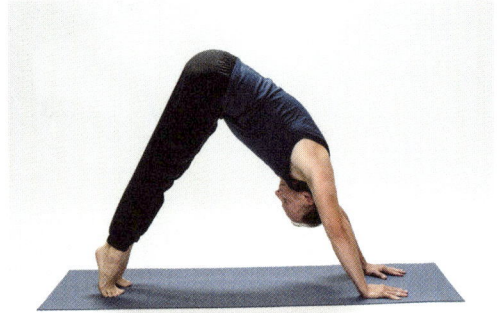

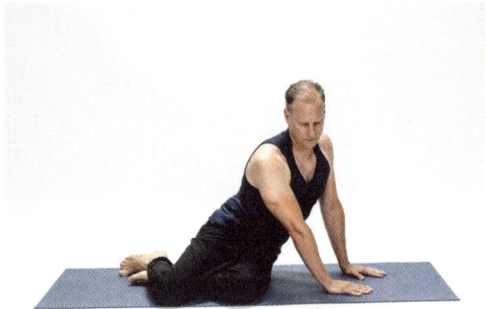

1. Sitting on your left glute, bend your knees, stack your legs and place your hands flat on the ground with your left hand slightly further forward than the right.

2. Exhale, round your back, lift onto your tippy toes and raise your hips and glutes to the ceiling. Straighten your legs.

3. Inhale and drop your hips while lifting your chest. Pull your shoulders back and down and expand your chest.

4. Exhale, tuck your chin and lift your hips and glutes towards the ceiling.

5. Inhale and lower to the starting position. Do 4–6 repetitions on each side.

Key Points

- Hollow out your abdominals and pull your navel to your spine when lifting your glutes skyward.

- Straighten your arms and legs as much as possible on the lifts.

- Squeeze your glutes and tops of the thighs on the hip drop position (Step 3) to release pressure on your low back. Lift off and land on the ground with control.

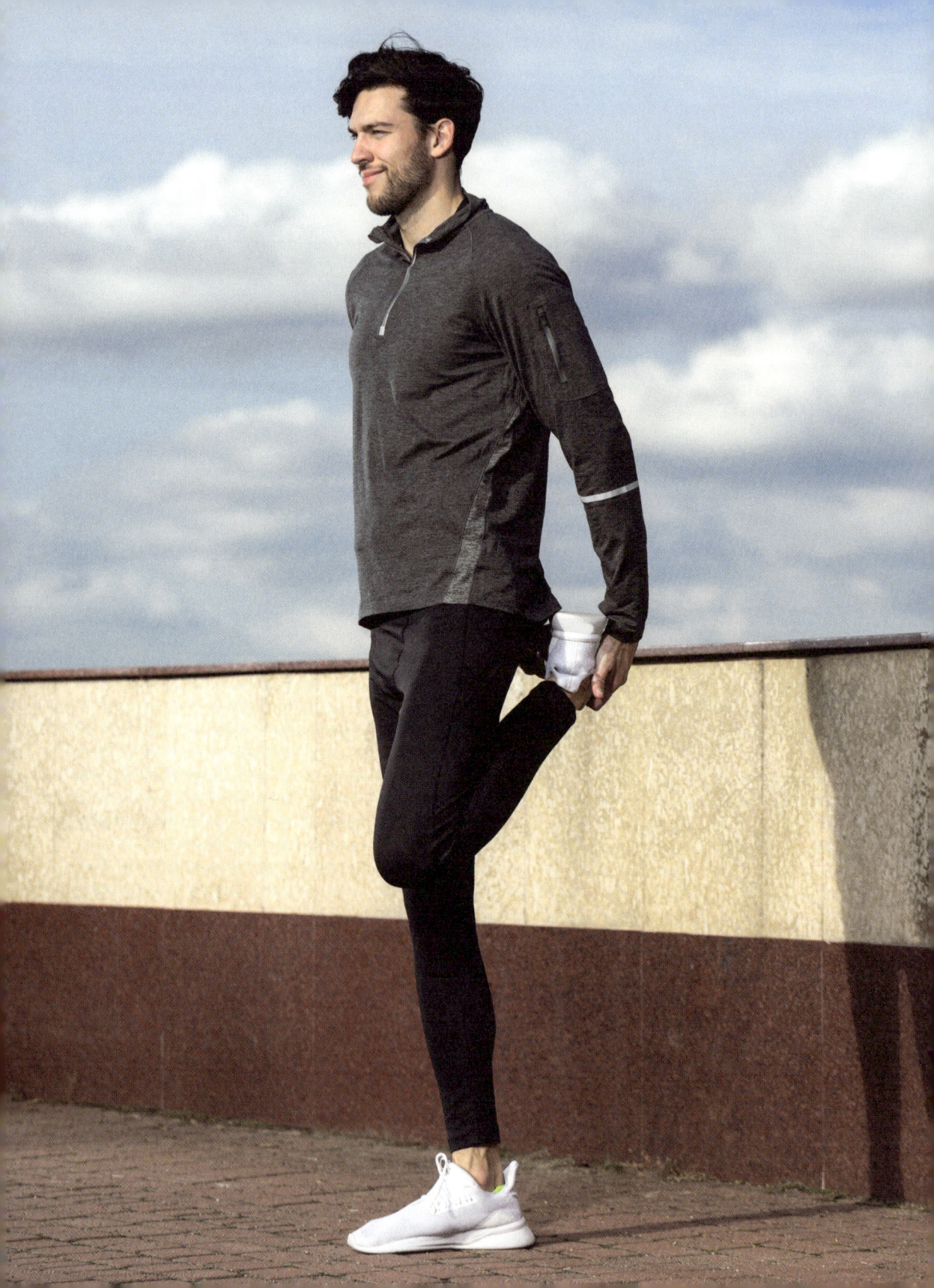

The Top 10 Stretches for Runners

Increase flexibility, reduce soreness, and recover faster with these runner-specific stretches.

CHILD'S POSE

AREAS TARGETED: Low back, spine, glutes, shoulders, hips

Soothe your back and catch your breath. My son does this pose with ease.

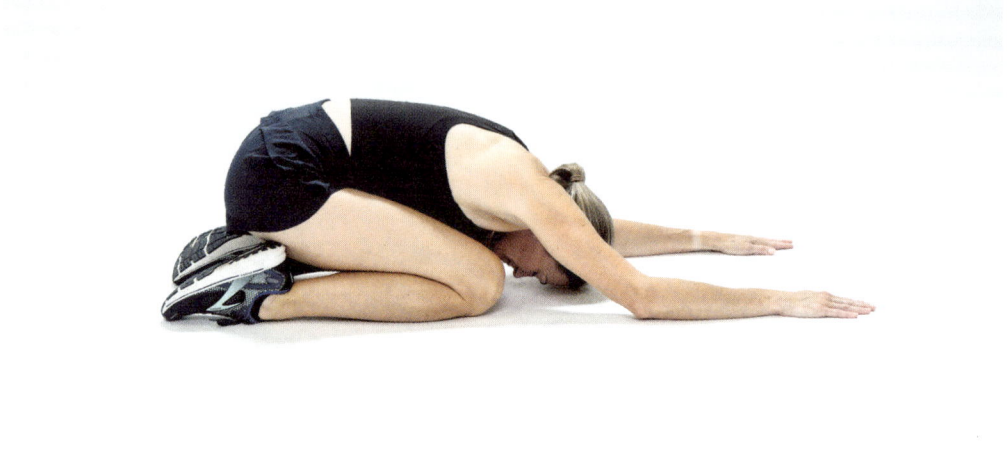

1. Place your knees hip-width apart on the floor and walk your hands forward as you sink your glutes back and down onto the heels.

2. Relax your shoulders back and release your forehead to the mat. You may also place your arms to your sides for less of a back and spine stretch. Square your hips and spread your fingers wide. Hold for 5–10 deep breaths and allow your body to completely relax.

Key Points

- Child's Pose is a wonderful pose for calming the mind and releasing the body through gentle yet profound stretching. It is easily accessible any time during your Pilates workouts when you need a moment to regroup, release and bring the focus back to your breath.

- Lengthen this pose by pressing your tailbone back and reaching your fingers forward while drawing your shoulders back and down. You may walk your hands further forward, lift your glutes slightly off your heels and sink your chest towards the floor in what is known as the Puppy Pose. This pose really enhances the natural curve in the spine and expands the shoulders.

- This is a huge favorite with my live classes and online videos. Whenever I mention it's time for Child's Pose, everyone collectively smiles, sighs and moves immediately into the pose. They don't need to be told twice, and neither will you.

◼ LUNGE

AREAS TARGETED: Hamstrings, quads and glutes

I love lunges of all kinds, but it's necessary to work on the foundation to ensure the best possible form.

1. Step your right foot forward so your knee is above your ankle. Extend the back leg by pressing the heel towards the floor. You may also bring that knee onto the mat.

2. Keeping your fingers on the mat, inhale and lift your arms up and back, exhale, sinking down into your legs. Do 5–10 breaths on each side.

Key Points

- Lunges build powerful core stability and flexibility while increasing balance.

- Lunges heat up your legs and glutes and helps to cultivate a strong focus on the movement.

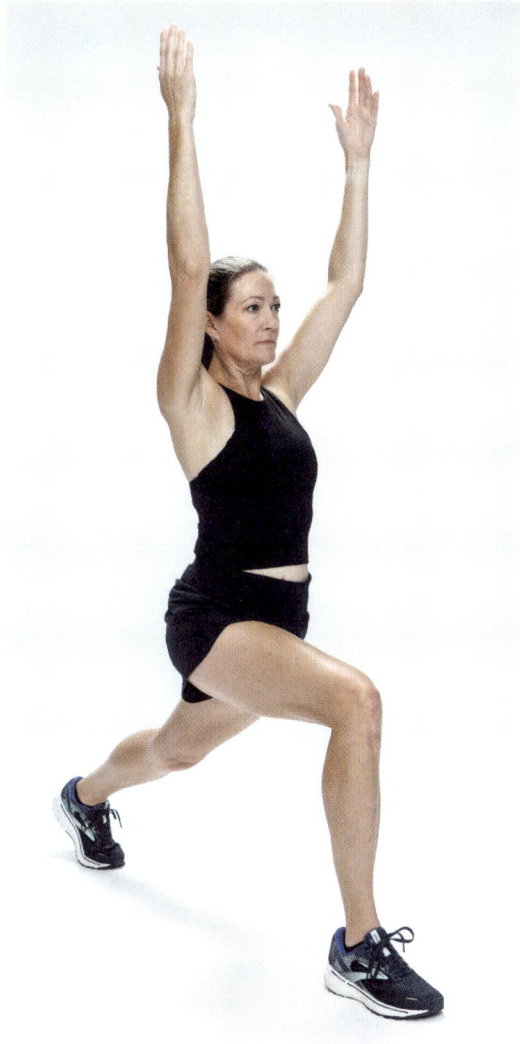

■ DOWNWARD FACING DOG

AREAS TARGETED: shoulders, hamstrings, calves, back, spine and glutes

This pose is the basis not only of my Power Yoga routines but also all other fitness disciplines I practice. All movements are easily accessible from Downward Facing Dog.

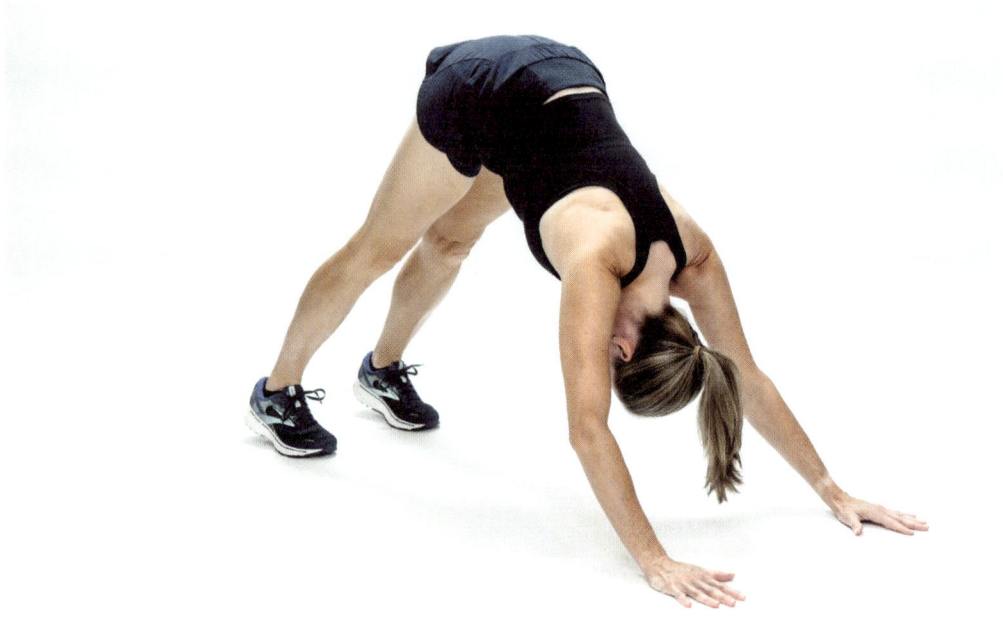

1. Bring your feet hip-width apart with the toes pointed forward. Keep a little softness in the knees and let your quads lengthen your legs.

2. Exhale, tuck your chin and fold forward from the hips, keeping softness in the knees. Lead with the top (crown) of the head.

3. Walk the hands forward until your body is in an upside-down "V" shape with your hands in front of your shoulders and feet behind the hips.

4. Spread your fingers wide to create a nice foundational base and draw weight off the wrists. Bring your hands shoulders-width and feet hip-width apart.

5. Exhale and sink back towards your heels, bringing them closer to the ground. Relax the shoulders and allow them to pull away from each other creating a nice stretch and allowing blood to flow in the upper back. Keep the chin tucked slightly and draw your nose towards the knees, tailbone up, heels down.

Key Points

- Downward Facing Dog is a stretch which drenches the body with energy and rejuvenates the mind. It stretches the shoulders, hamstrings, calves, back, spine and glutes…and it feels really good the deeper you delve into the pose.

- The inversion factor in Down Dog also has a calming effect as fresh blood is drawn into the head and brain, helping to center the mind and thoughts.

- It's a stretch and strengthening pose which challenges both mind and body together, creating a total training experience in just one pose.

UPWARD FACING DOG

AREAS TARGETED: Glutes, spine, back, chest, shoulders, triceps and hips

Open the flexibility in your back and spine with these backbends.

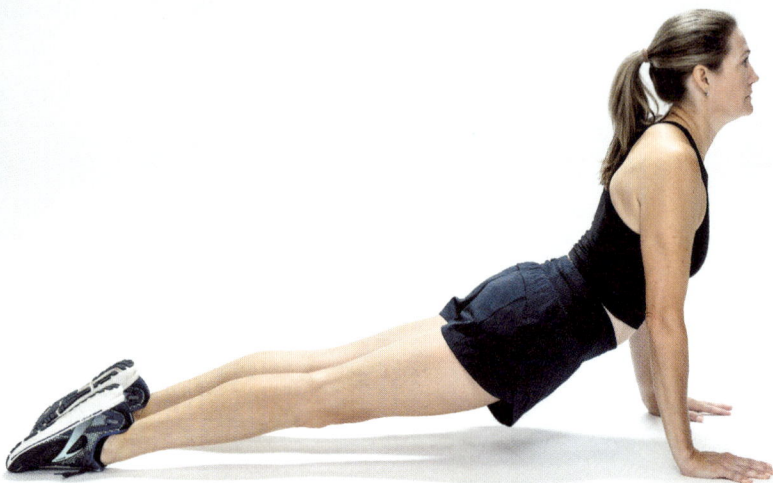

1. Lie on your stomach and place your hands under your shoulders with your elbows hugging the ribs. Extend your legs behind you with the tops of your feet on the mat.

2. Inhale and lift the upper body so your arms are straight (with a tiny bit of softness in the elbows). Draw your shoulders back and down and expand your chest. Squeeze your glutes and quads and lift your legs and knees off the mat. Hold for 5–10 deep breaths.

Key Points

- Holding this pose really strengthens the upper body. You receive the benefits of stretching and strengthening in one pose.

- This pose allows for much better and more open breathing, so make sure your shoulders are down and your chest is opening and expanding. It might feel very strange to open your chest like this if you're used to having shoulders which roll forward all day, but it's essential. Proper posture will encourage maximum oxygen flow.

- If you're someone who spends many hours in a seated or deep squat position, this pose will bring mobility to your back and hips while lifting your overall posture.

BUTTERFLY

AREAS TARGETED: Inner thighs, hips, groin, hamstrings and knees

This is a wonderful stretch for opening your hips.

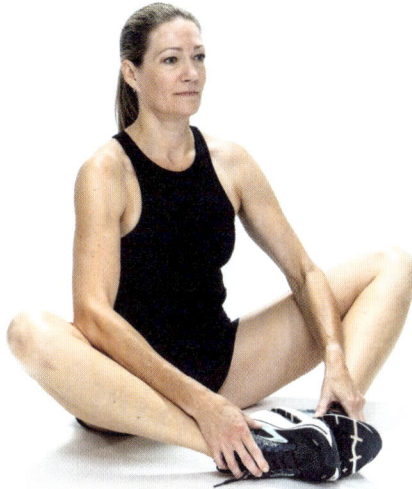

1. Begin seated, bend your knees and bring the soles of your feet together. Sit up tall, roll your shoulders back and down and expand your chest.

2. Place your hands on your ankles or feet and pry your hips open by placing your elbows on your legs while hinging forward. Hold for 10–15 breaths.

Key Points

- Continue pressing your knees down with your elbows and hinging forward from the hips with each exhale.

- To reduce stress on your knees, move your feet forward. Increase the intensity of the stretch by bringing the knees closer.

- Avoid rounding your back and focus on lengthening from the hips to the crown of the head.

PIGEON

AREAS TARGETED: Hips, back, glutes and shoulders

One of the most beloved stretches and a mid-level popularity bird.

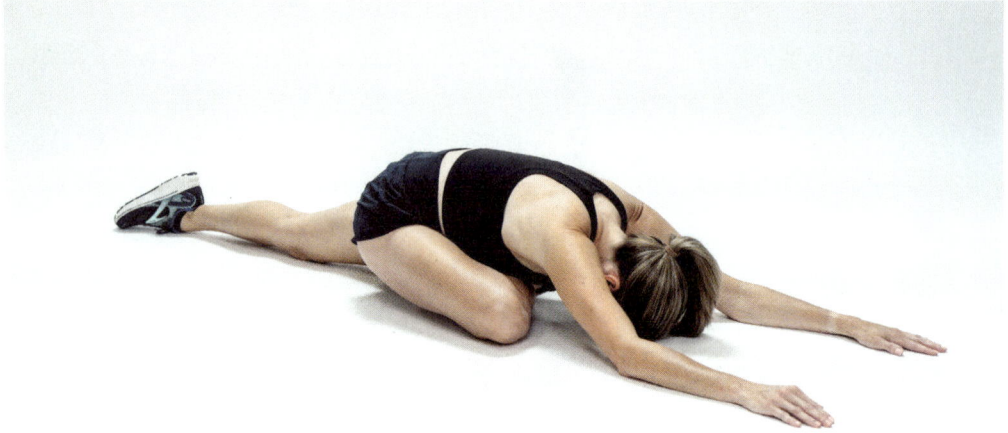

1. From Downward Facing Dog (page 102), exhale and bring your right knee forward and onto the ground. Place your hands under your shoulders and lift tall as you square your hips, slide your left leg back and open your right leg. Place your weight right over the center of the pose and walk your hands forward. Release your upper body and soak up this beautiful stretch. Hold for 10–15 breaths on each side.

Key Points

- Your hips store up so much tension, tightness and stress that it affects the rest of your body. Pigeon pose is legendary for unlocking the hips and the surrounding area. Practicing it every day will bring more mobility and release.

- As you add more Pigeon to your training, walk your front foot forward as your body allows. The goal is to bring your front leg into a right angle for optimum knee, hip, glute and back release.

- Practice holding Proud Pigeon first, with hands on the mat and lifting the upper body while sinking your shoulders back and down and expanding your chest. Feel the added stretch in your abdominals and chest. You will also receive a nice contraction in your shoulders and triceps.

FIGURE FOUR

AREAS TARGETED: Hips, glutes, lower back

A staple for all serious stretching routines.

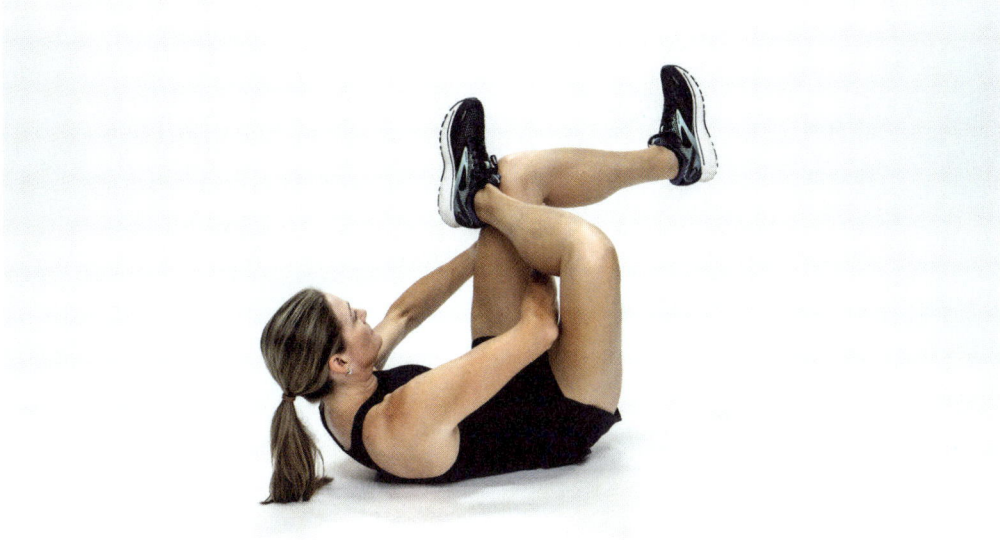

1. Lie on your back, bend your left knee, place your left foot flat on the ground and place your right ankle on top of your left thigh.

2. Reach your right arm in between your legs and your left arm around the outside. Lace your fingers together on the back of your left leg.

3. Exhale and pull your legs towards you, using your right elbow to press into your right leg to further open the stretch. The head and shoulder may come off the mat if you wish. Pump 5–10 breaths into this stretch and repeat on both sides.

Key Points

- This is a fantastic stretch for relief from intense squat, crouch and lunge training.
- The closer you place your grounded foot to your glutes, the more intense the stretch. You may extend your other leg to the sky for an extra hamstring stretch.
- Actively pull your legs closer with each exhale and sway slightly side to side to target your hip and glute muscles deeper.

SPIDER

AREAS TARGETED: Hamstrings and calves

The Spider is a frozen Single Straight Leg Stretch (page 30) designed to expand and lengthen your hamstrings.

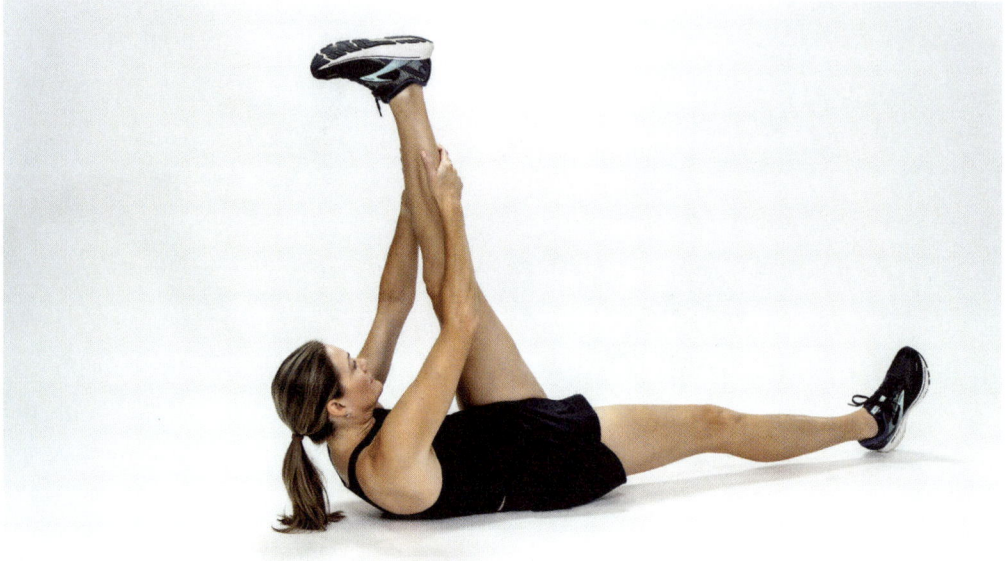

1. Lie on your back and extend your right leg to the sky. Lengthen your left leg in front of you on the floor. Grab your right leg on the ankle, calf or hamstring and lengthen further and lift your head, neck and shoulders off the mat as you exhale.

2. Inhale, bend your right knee slightly and exhale further into the stretch. Bring your nose towards your knee and flex the elevated foot with each exhale.

Key Points

- Keep your elbows pointed to the outside so you have more space to maneuver deeper into the stretch.
- Keep your hips square.
- When bringing your nose towards your knee, lift with your abdominals, not your neck and head.

LYING SPINAL TWIST

AREAS TARGETED: Spine, back, glutes, and chest

Everyone enjoys and benefits greatly from this life-changing twist.

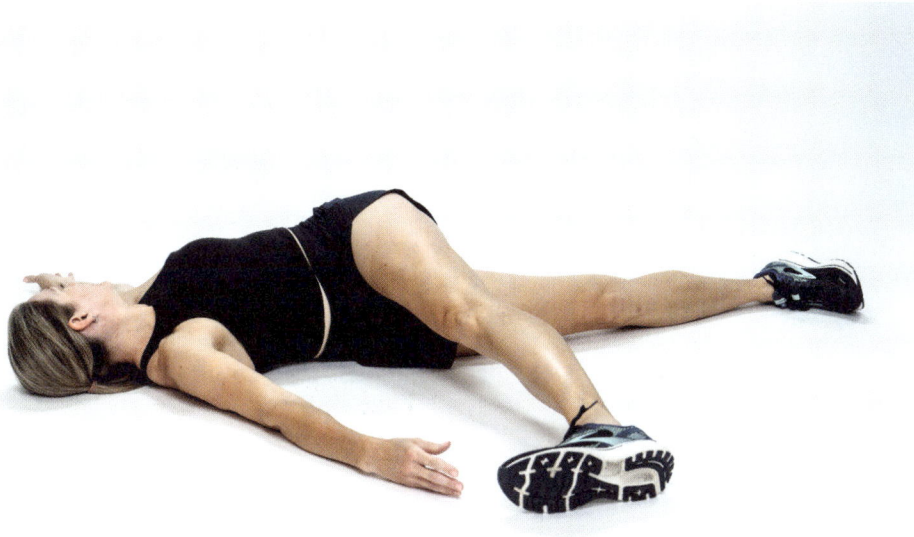

1. From Spider (page 108) either bend the top left leg and draw it across your body or go directly into the twist with your left leg extended.

2. Exhale and use your hands to help guide your leg to the floor safely and effectively. Rotate your upper body to the left and sink your shoulder towards or into the floor. Turn your face to your left hand. Hold on each side for 10–15 breaths.

Key Points

- Continue lengthening your leg across with your exhales. Grasp your foot or ankle with the hand that's closest and pull your foot higher.

- This stretch decompresses the spine, stretches the back and glutes, and realigns the spine. It also opens the chest, calms the mind and encourages fresh blood flow to the digestive organs.

- This stretch is also a great stress reliever, both mental and physical. Move yourself out of the way of the twist and allow it to deepen with your breaths. Relax. Release. Renew.

KNEES TO CHEST

AREAS TARGETED: Lower back, glutes, quad, knees, hamstrings and spinal flexibility

Our final cooldown stretch is an ode to lower back release and regeneration.

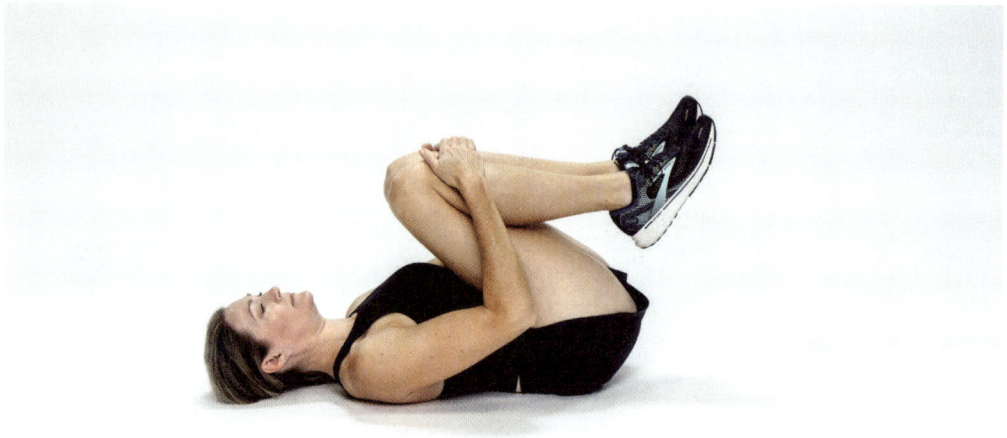

1. Lie on your back and pull your knees to your chest. Place your hands on your knees and gently pull them and the tops of your thighs into your chest.

2. Relax your head on the mat and relax your feet and ankles. Rock your knees gently side-to-side after holding the pose for 10–15 breaths. Let go and allow the pose to release and move naturally.

Key Points

- This stretch is a wonderful meditative experience. You will feel your low back massaging gently into the mat and the knees stretching and releasing.

- Keep your knees together while drawing them into your chest. This will increase the stretch to your quads and knees.

- For a more intense version of this stretch, bend your knees and lift your feet. Smoosh your thighs into your chest while holding your ankles. The tops of the feet point to the sky.

CHAPTER 4

Run Strong: Core, Balance & Stability Training

Alright runners, the lights are on and it's showtime! We've talked the talk, now it's time to put these powerhouse Pilates exercises into motion and start running faster, smoother, and stronger in real time.

You might be asking: "Why do I need core strength, balance, and stability workouts?" Great question. Read this, and then do the workouts. That's where the magic happens. Once you hit the mat, don't look back.

Let's start with the **core**. Pilates core strength is the secret weapon every runner needs in their arsenal. It beautifully stabilizes your body, helping you maintain fluid running form, strong posture, and consistent alignment with every stride. Less flailing, more flowing. A rock-solid core reduces excess movement, boosts posture, and turns your upper-to-lower body energy transfer into a well-oiled running machine. And you know what? That core power also helps protect you from the usual issues—nagging injuries in the spine, hips, pelvis, and joints. Say goodbye to breakdowns. Say hello to breakthrough runs.

Now let's talk **balance**. A client once told me that running is basically "a workout made of thousands of awkward one-legged hops" and honestly, it's a perfect description. That's why balance training is *so* critical. It helps you stay tall, aligned, and efficient, especially when you're tired or pounding through uneven terrain. And let's face it: better balance = fewer wipeouts and way more energy saved.

Now you might be asking, what's the deal with **stability**? It's the glue that holds it all together. Stability is your body's ability to keep those joints—hips, knees, ankles—steady and secure through motion. It's what keeps your form strong when everything else wants to give up. With Pilates, we build powerful stabilizers—core, glutes, hip muscles—that absorb shock, keep your form clean, and help you run long, strong, and injury-free.

These dynamic Pilates flows are loaded with challenging, energizing exercises designed to build balance from the inside out and help your body stabilize through anything—running, jogging, sprinting, power walking, you name it.

Practice each flow several times, and focus on deep breathing, precise movement, and smooth transitions from one move to the next. I call them "flows" because that's exactly how they should feel—fluid, controlled, and powerful, like water in motion.

You'll get more results in less time and feel like you're unlocking new levels of performance with every session. So remember, quality over quantity. Every rep counts when you're training like a pro.

Note: Use these exercises as part of your school athletic training, whether it's for PE, track/cross country, all the major sports or even homeroom classes. Pilates works wonders for Kindergartners up to high school. All you need is a few minutes to make a huge difference in your running and athletic performance.

Let's flow, let's move, let's run like never before.

I know a lot of runners. I know they are not big fans of long, tedious workouts. They want quick, effective and easily accessible flows that will do the job in a short amount of time. That's what these are. Want a longer flow? Repeat them, do more repetitions or perform the exercises slower, squeezing every drop of pliability and core strength out of each one.

Flow #1: Core Workout for Stability

Fire it up!

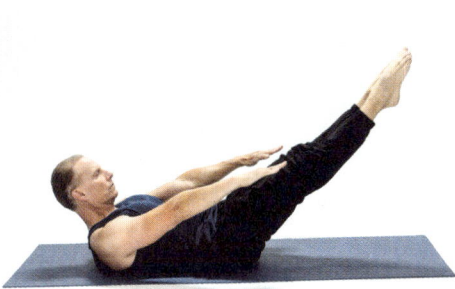

Pilates 100

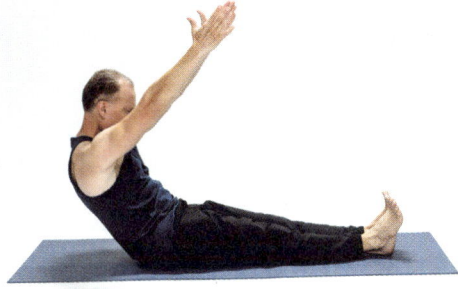

Roll Up

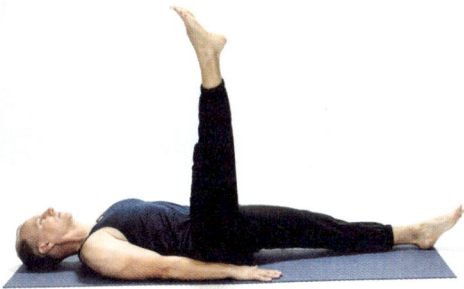

One Leg Circles

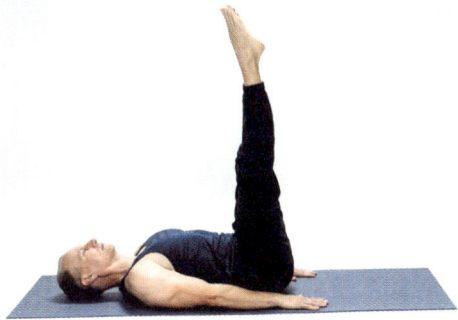

Corkscrew

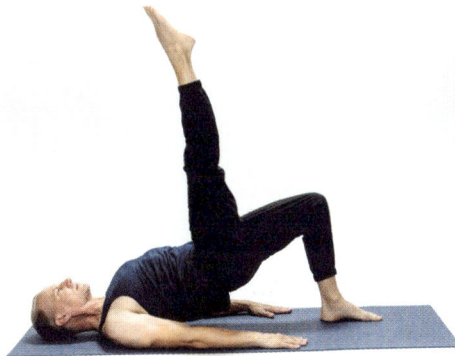

Shoulder Bridge

Flow #2: Pre-Run Stability Workout

Set the tone for a great run!

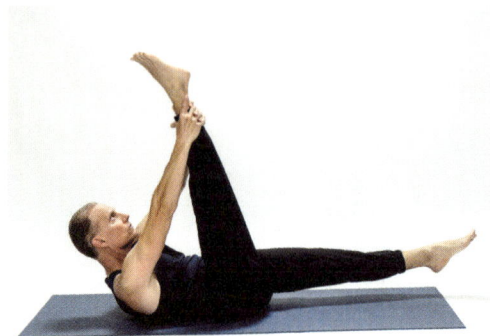

Single Straight Leg Stretch

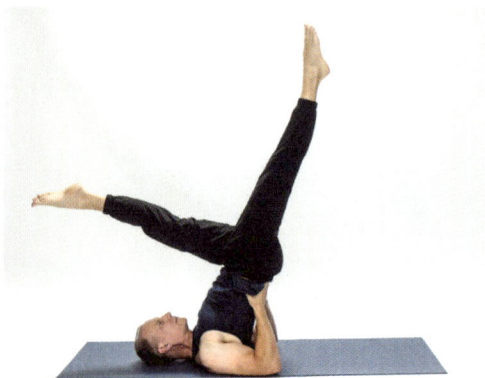

Scissors

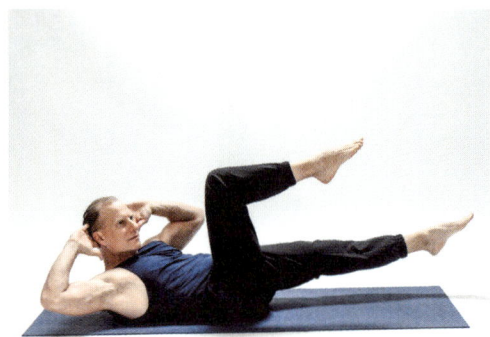

Criss Cross

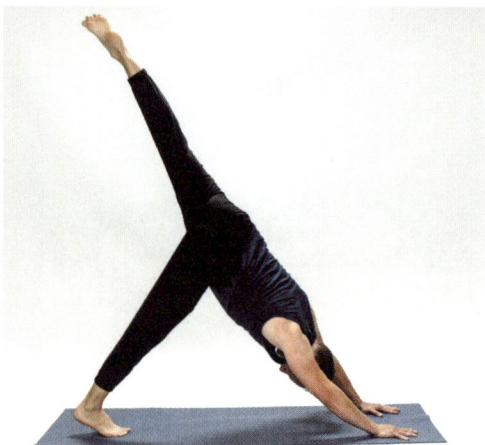

Down Dog Leg Lifts

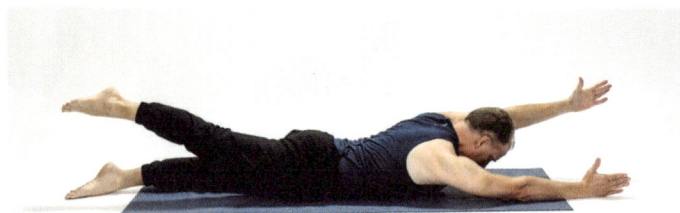

Swimming

Flow #3: Pilates Workout for Balance

Run with balance and precision.

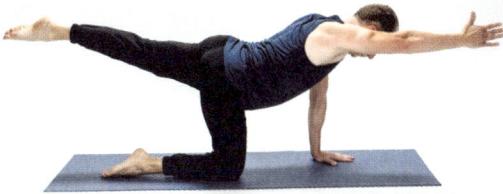

Birddog

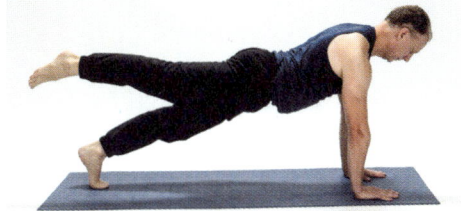

Leg Pull Front

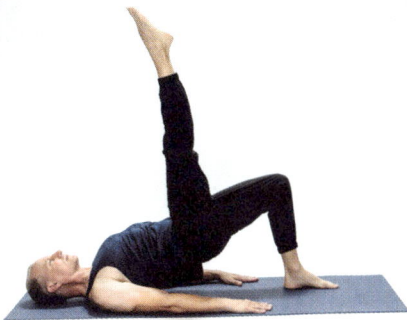

Shoulder Bridge

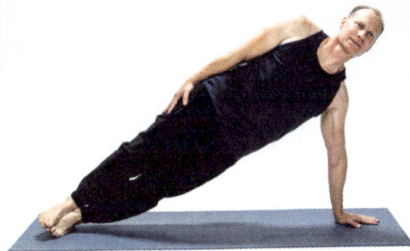

Star

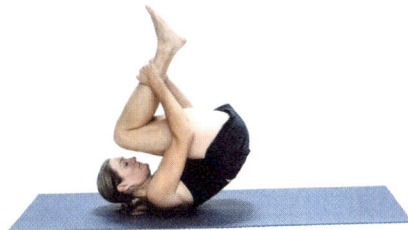

Rolling like a Ball

Flow #4: Pre-Run Ab Activator

Set a fire in your abs to carry you through a blistering run.

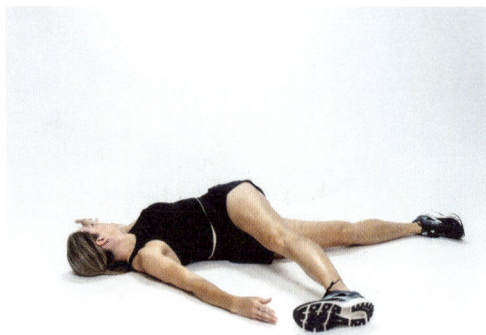

Lying Spinal Twist

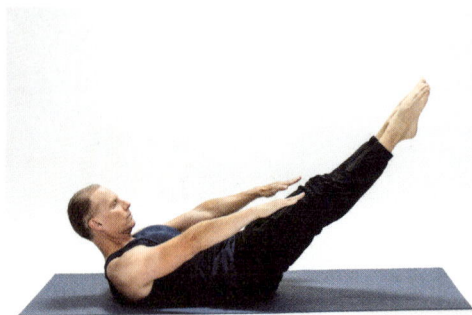

Pilates 100

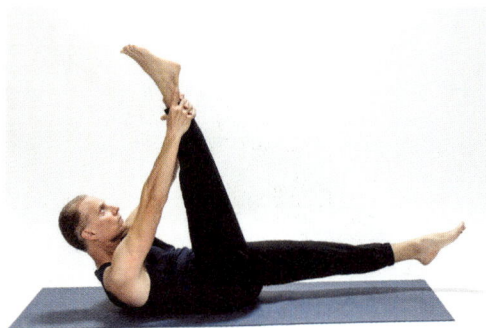

Single Straight Leg Stretch

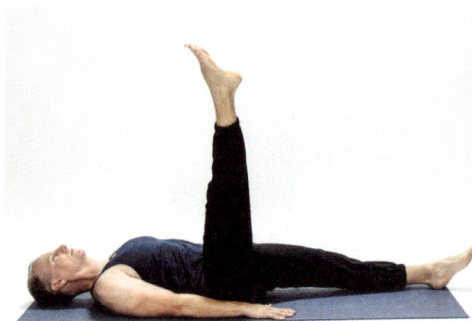

One Leg Circles

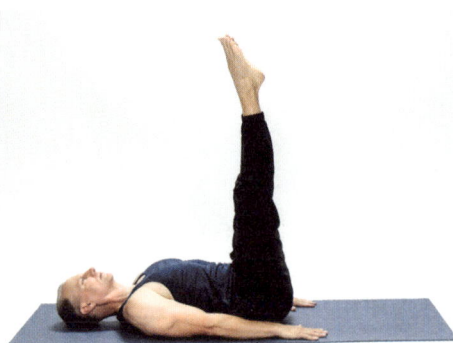

Corkscrew

Flow #5: Core Stability Activator

Build a strong, balanced core to absorb those thousands of heel strikes.

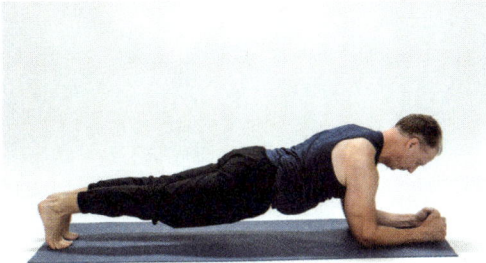

Forearm Plank

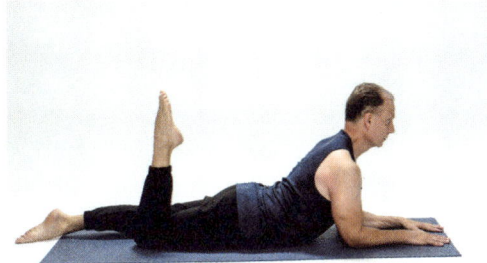

Single Leg Kick

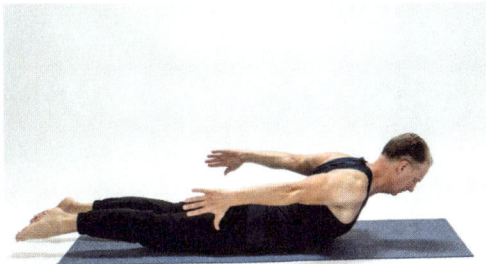

Double Leg Kick

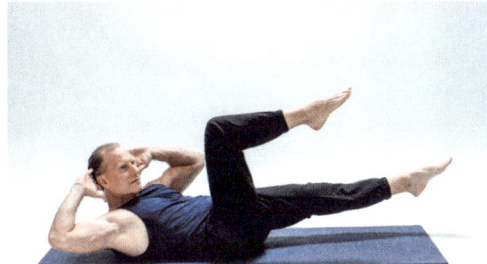

Criss Cross

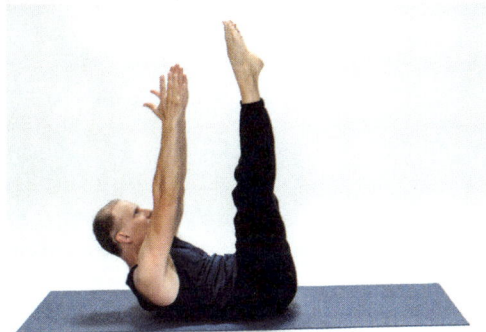

Backstroke

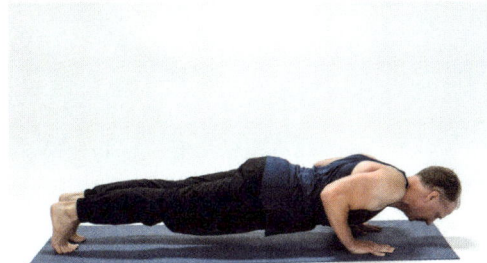

Pilates Push-Ups

Flow #5: Core Stability Activator (continued)

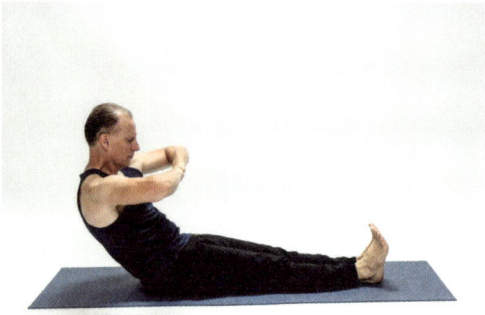

Rowing from the Sternum

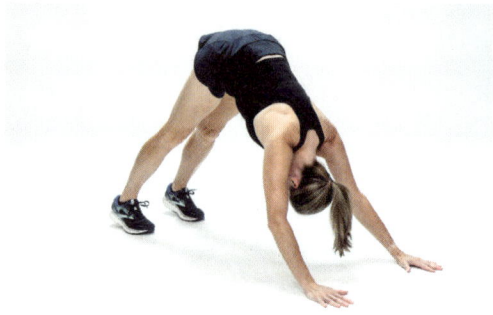

Downward Facing Dog

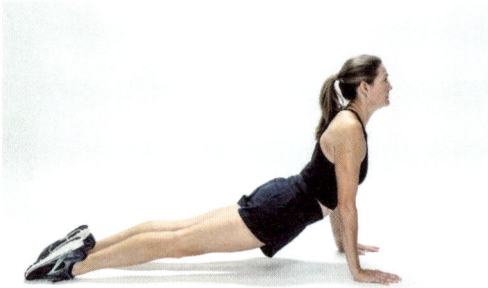

Upward Facing Dog

CHAPTER 5

Flexibility, Mobility & Leg Training for Runners

Welcome to your flow workouts! Each one in this chapter is laser-focused on boosting two superhero skills: flexibility (think smooth, full-range muscle movement) and mobility (controlled, powerful, joint-friendly action). When these two join forces, you get a body that moves better, feels looser, and stays injury-free. That's what I call a winning combo!

Now let's talk about your legs—the MVPs of your running game. Can a runner hit peak performance with tight, weak, unbalanced legs? (Spoiler alert: nope!) Whether you're a weekend warrior or training for your next marathon, strong, supple, and stable legs are absolutely essential for success.

That's why I've included one of my all-time favorites: the classic Side Leg Series. I've led thousands of runners and athletes through this routine, and the feedback is always the same—stronger legs, tighter cores, and a playlist of satisfying grunts and groans with a dollop of cursing. Get ready to feel the burn and love the results. It's go time!

Craving a longer workout? No problem! Just repeat the flow, slow it down, or crank up the reps. The secret is in the control—squeeze every ounce of mobility, strength, and core power from each move. Short on time? No excuses. These flows are your new secret weapon. Let's go!

Flow #1: Hip Stretch, Release & Opening Sequence

Open your hips and improve mobility, injury prevention and efficiency of your strides.

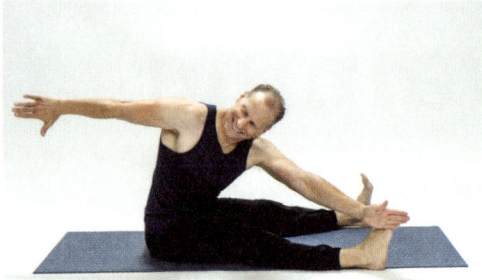

Saw

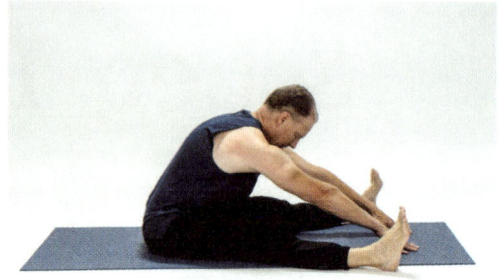

Spine Stretch

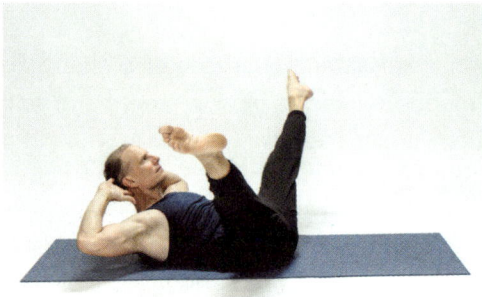

Straddle Crunch

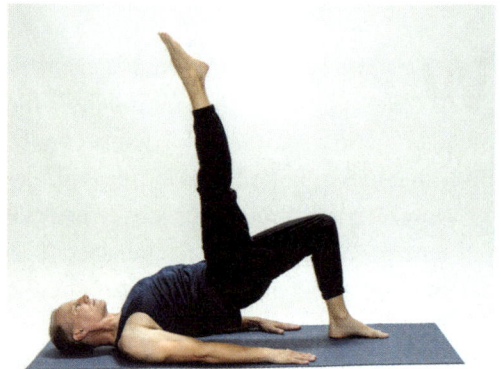

Shoulder Bridge

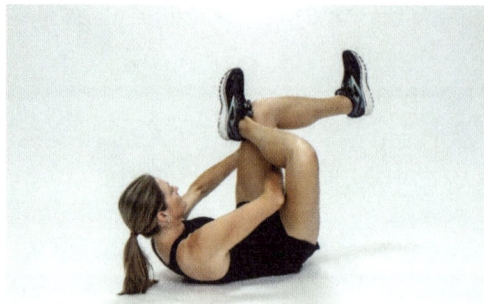

Figure Four

Flow #2: Rowing & Side Leg

Just as it says: dive into the seldom seen or practiced powerful Pilates Rowing series and top it off with the brutally fun and effective Side Leg Series.

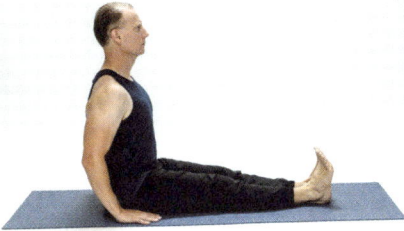

Rowing from the Hips

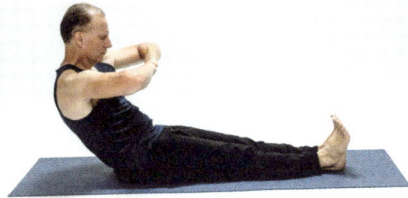

Rowing from the Sternum

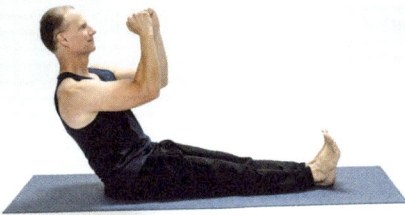

Rowing 90 Degrees

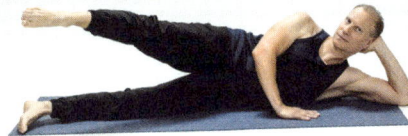

Circles (both sides)

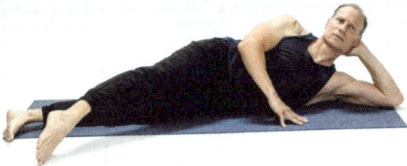

Taps (both sides)

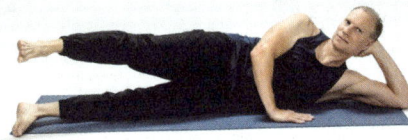

Kicks (both sides)

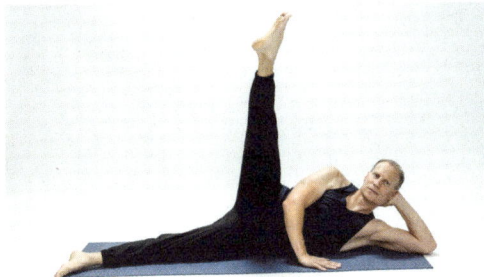

Kick Ups (both sides)

Flow #3: Pre-Run Core & Hamstring Activator

Loosen up your hamstrings and fire your core with these exercises designed to help you run faster, smoother and with less tension.

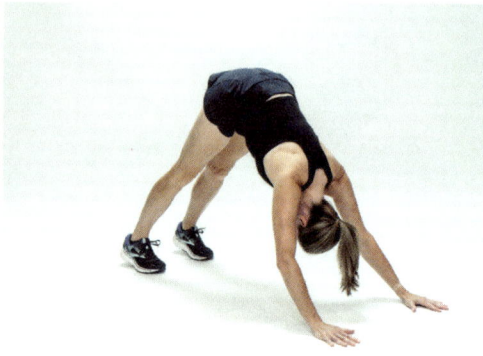

Downward Facing Dog

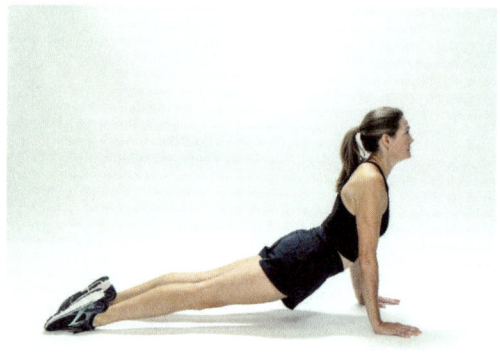

Upward Facing Dog

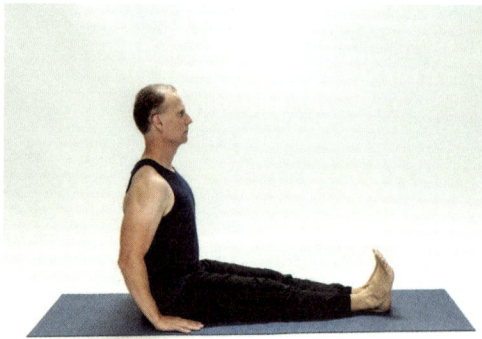

Rowing from the Hips

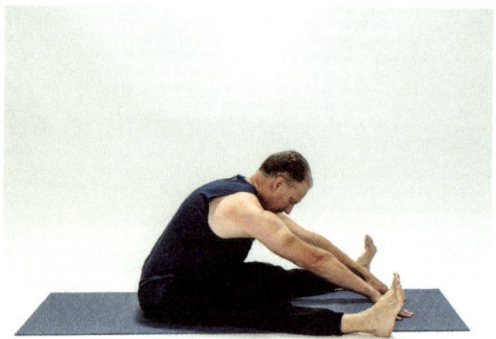

Spine Stretch

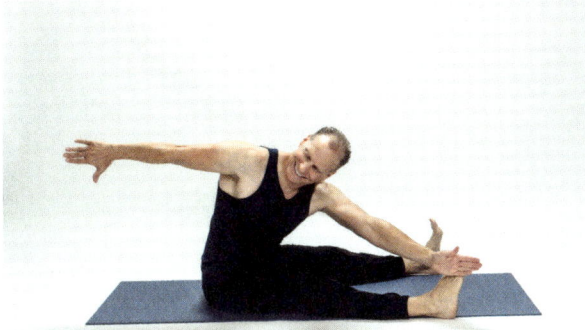

Saw

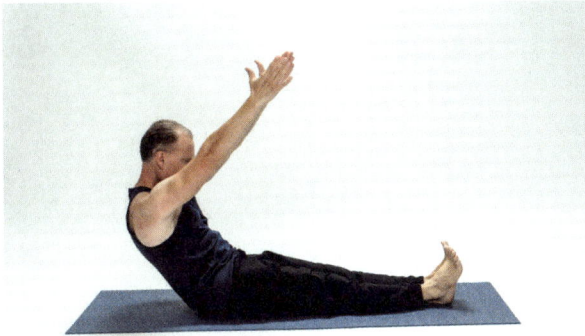

Roll Up

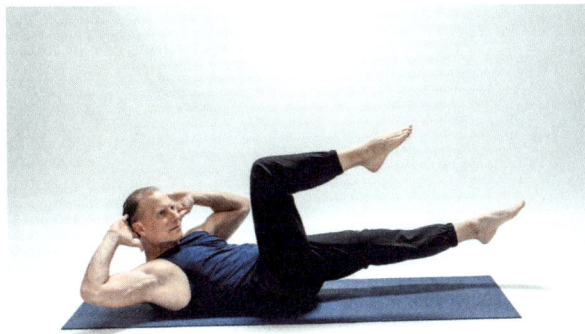

Criss Cross

Flow #4: Mobility & Flexibility Pilates Workout

Do this flow anytime you want to boost your core strength and massively increase your body's flexibility and mobility.

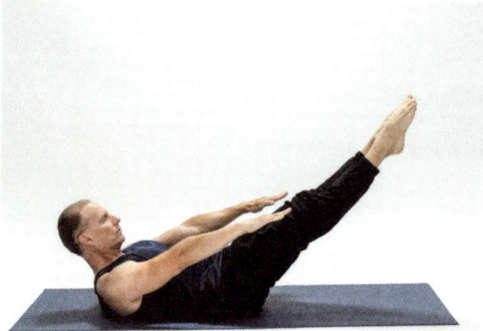

Pilates 100

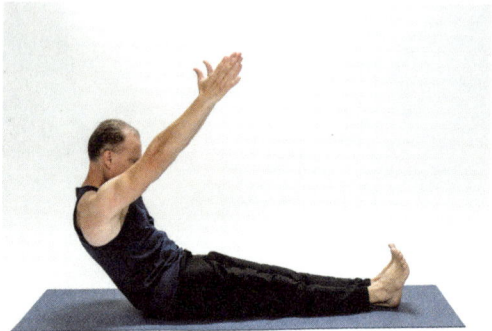

Roll Up

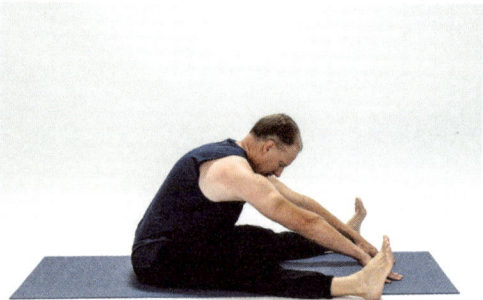

Spine Stretch

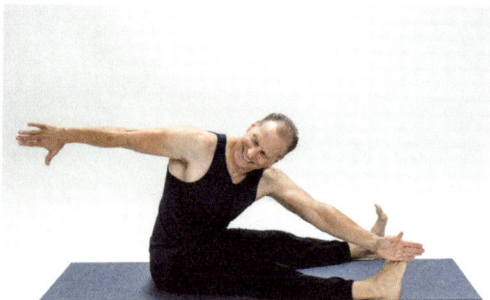

Saw

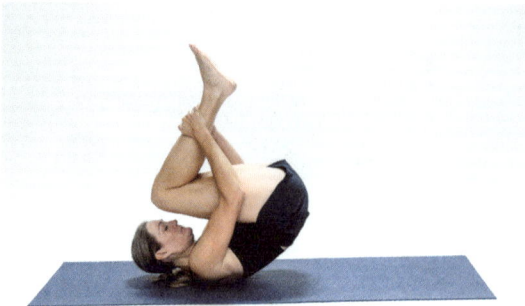

Rolling like a Ball

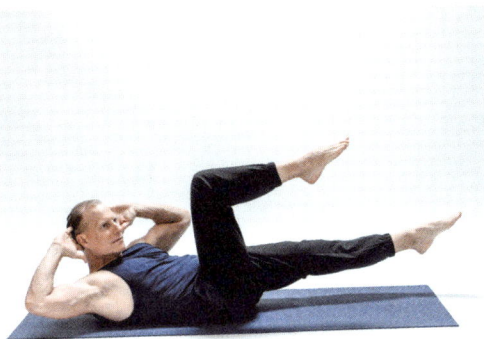

Criss Cross

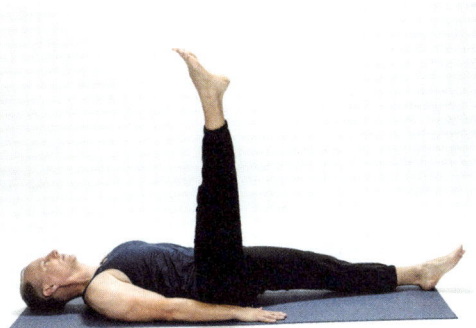

One Leg Circles

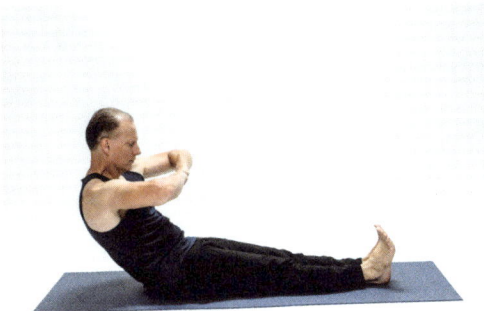

Rowing from the Sternum

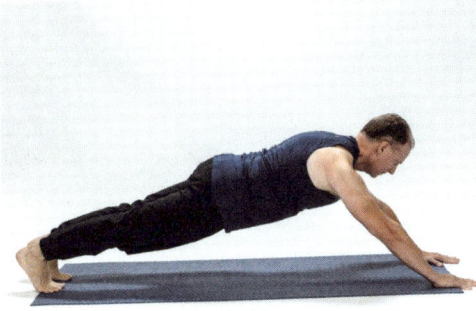

Elephant Plank

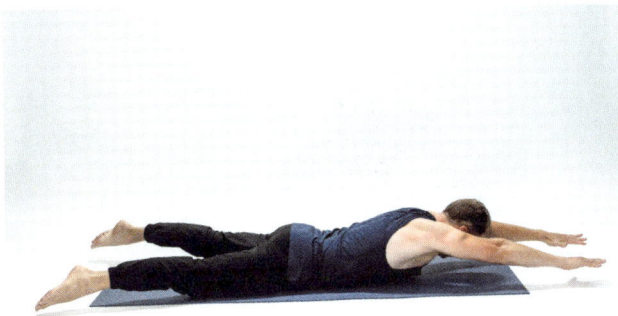

Pulling the Straps

Flow #4: Mobility & Flexibility Pilates Workout (continued)

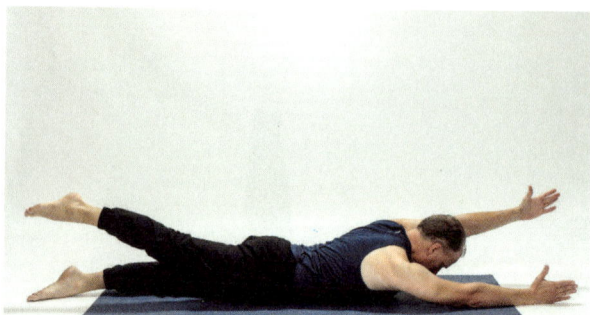

Swimming

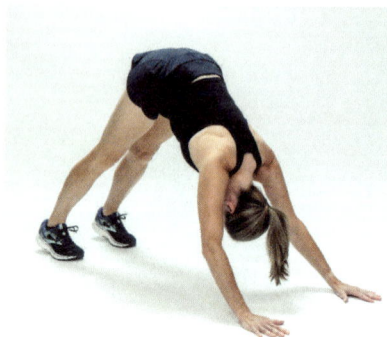

Downward Facing Dog

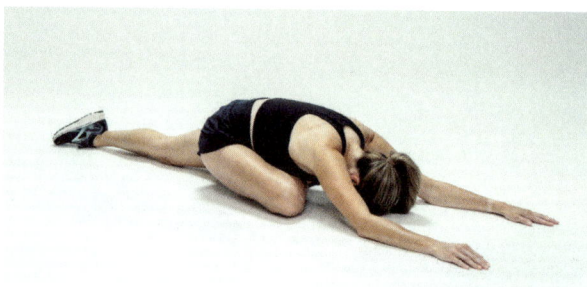

Pigeon

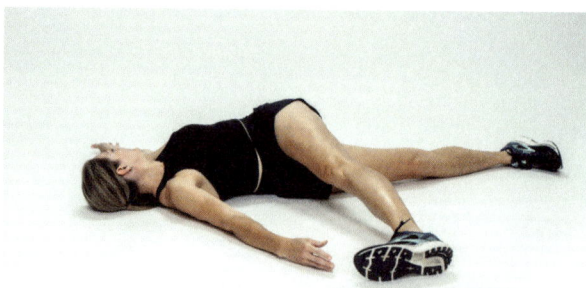

Lying Spinal Twist

CHAPTER 6

Injury Prevention, Warm-Up, Cool Down & Recovery

Maybe you've been training intensely but still feel like you're stuck and your body isn't responding the way you want. Nagging injuries, tight muscles, imbalances, or just that heavy, sluggish feeling can drag you down. But take a deep breath (seriously, do it now!) because help is on the way.

These flows are all about *recovery*, my friend. We're talking long, delicious stretches, tension-releasing moves, and techniques to help your body come back stronger than ever. Recovery isn't optional, it's essential. Without it, you're heading warp speed into a brick wall (and nobody wants that).

So, make these flows your daily ritual. Breathe deep—10 to 20 slow, mindful breaths per stretch ought to do it. Focus deep, tune in, and treat your body like the high-performance machine it is and can be. The more presence you bring, the better your runs will feel. This is your time. Treat it as such.

These flows are the heart and soul of this book. They're your secret weapon for running stronger, smoother, and smarter as long as you keep showing up. So hit the mat, breathe deep, and let's make every aspect of your running feel like magic!

Flow #1: Post Run Recovery Stretch

Finish your run in style.

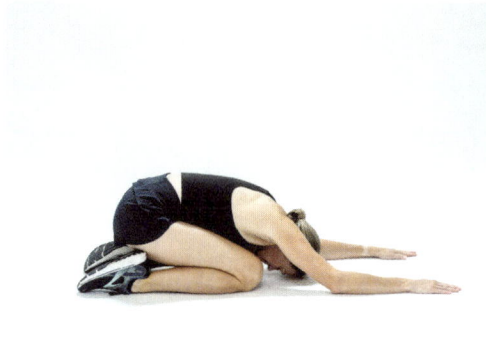

Child's Pose

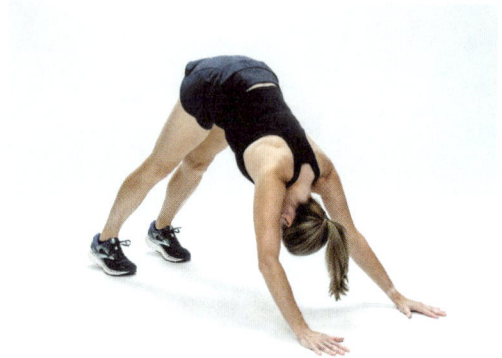

Downward Facing Dog

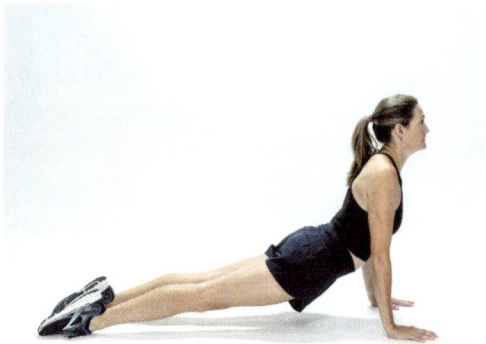

Upward Facing Dog

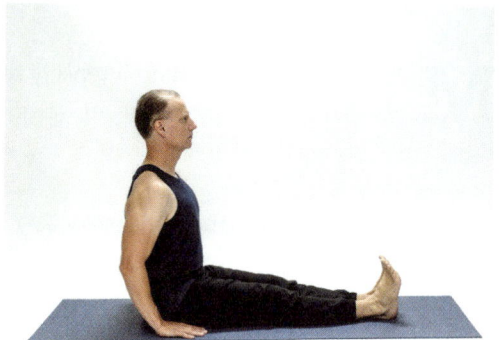

Rowing from the Hips

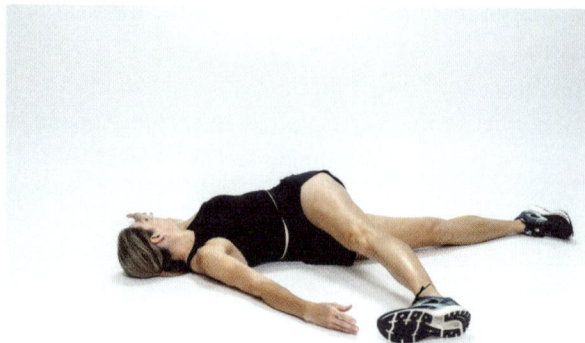

Lying Spinal Twist

Flow #2: Hips & Low Back Release

Your hips and low back will breathe a sigh of relief.

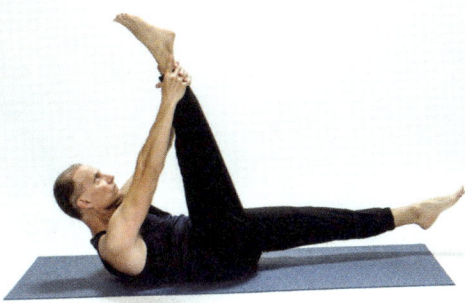

Single Straight Leg Stretch

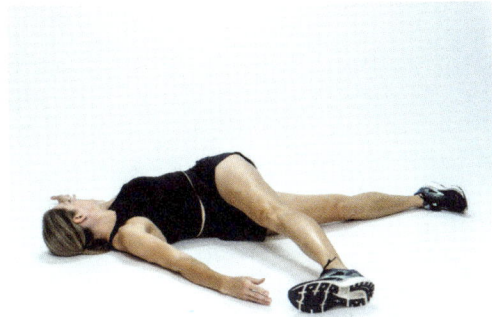

Lying Spinal Twist

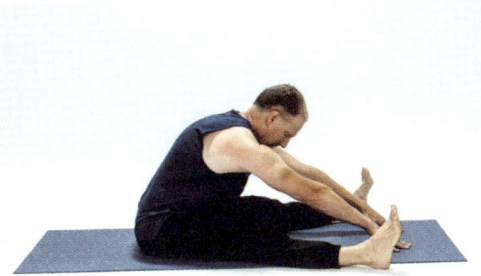

Spine Stretch

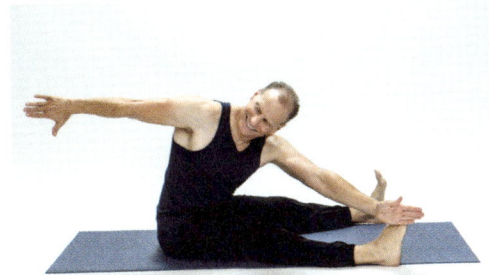

Saw

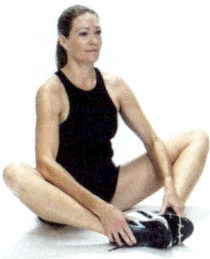

Butterfly

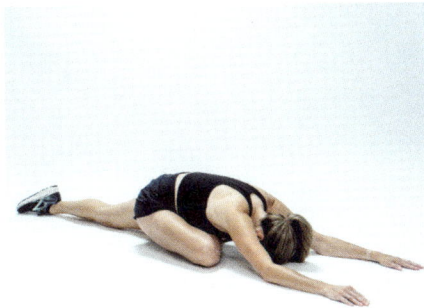

Pigeon

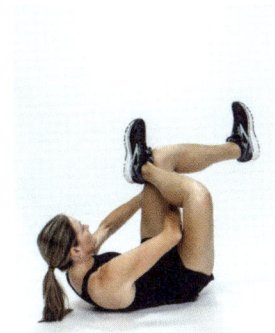

Figure Four

Flow #3: Warm Up Flow

Plan (run) for success with this delicious warm up flow.

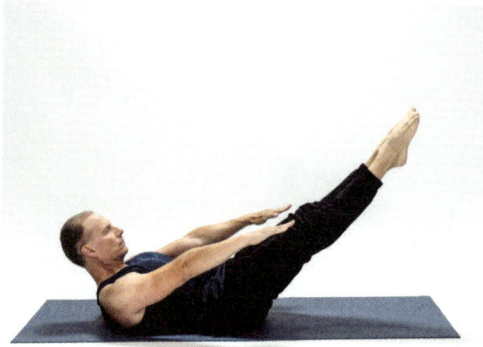
Pilates 100

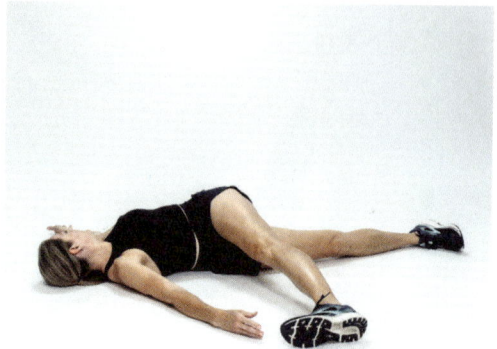
Lying Spinal Twist

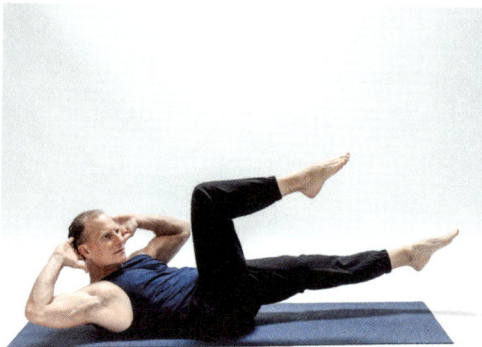
Criss Cross

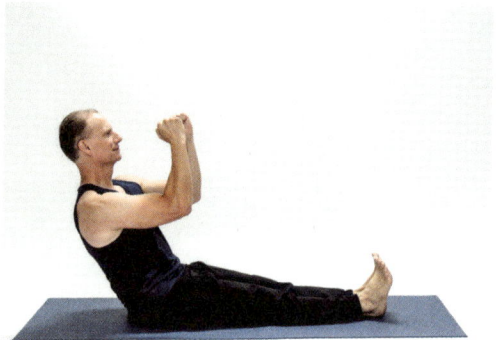
Rowing 90 Degrees

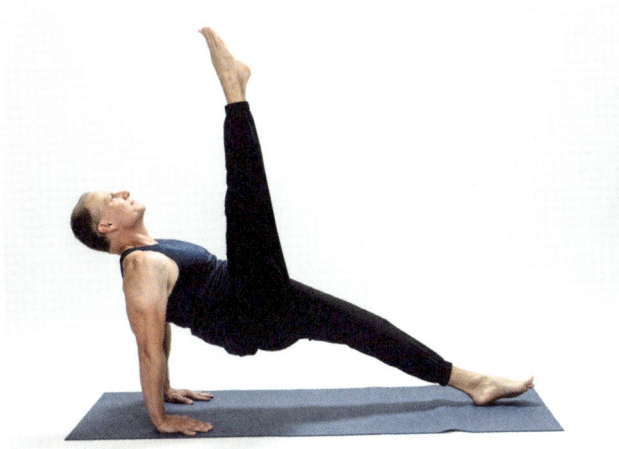

Leg Pull

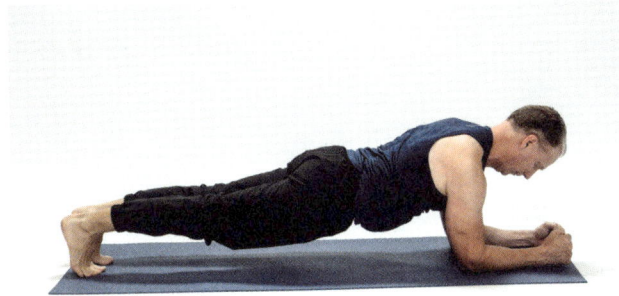

Forearm Plank

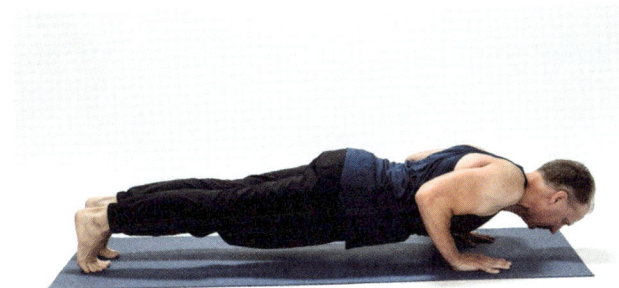

Pilates Push-Ups

Flow #4: Cool Down Flow

Looking to completely release mind, body and spirit after your run? You've come to the right flow.

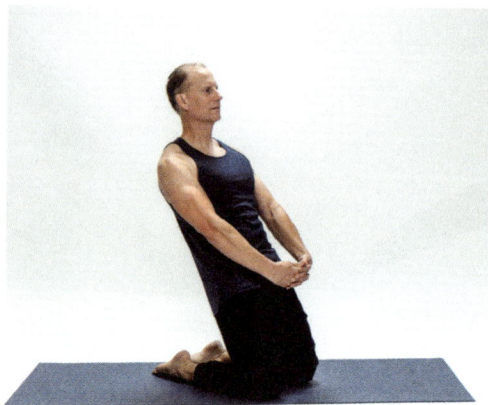

Camel Pulse

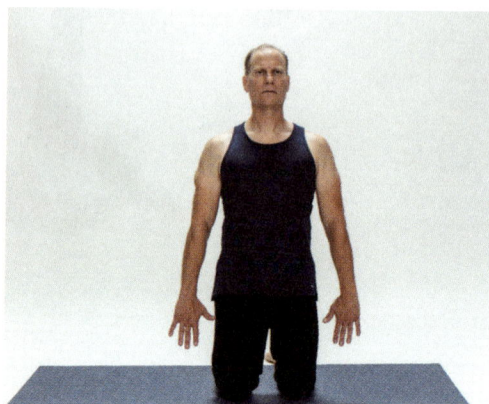

Chest Expansion

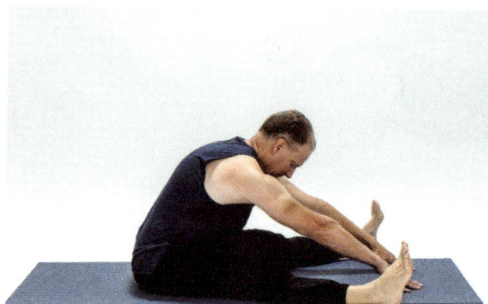

Spine Stretch

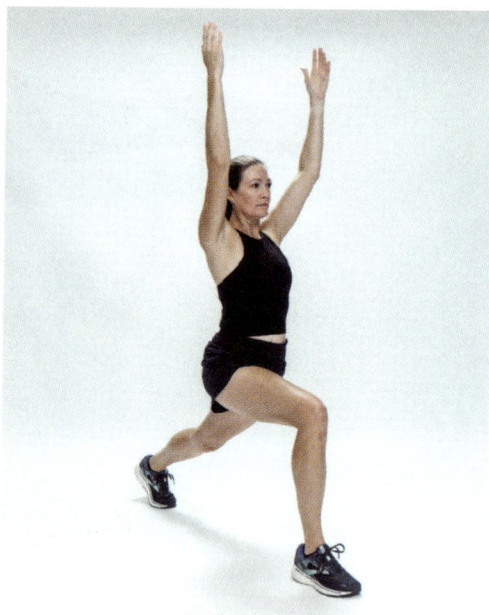

Lunge

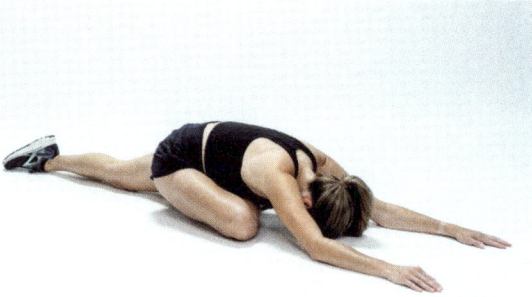

Pigeon

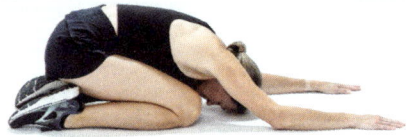

Child's Pose

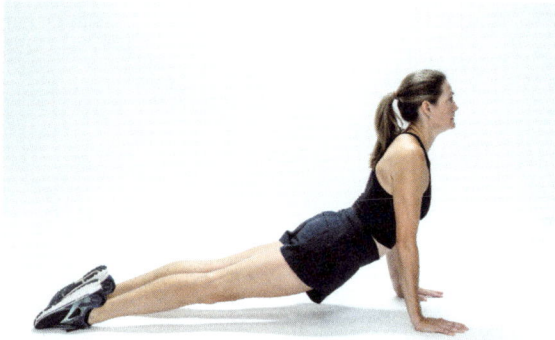

Upward Facing Dog

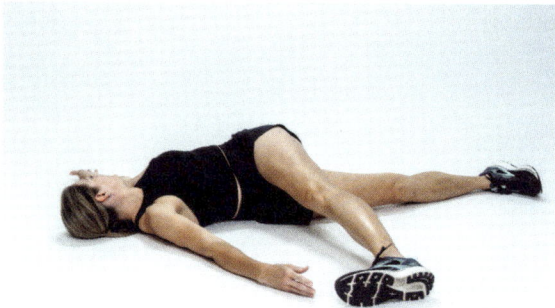

Lying Spinal Twist

Flow #5: Injury Prevention Routine

Run longer, better and faster with less nagging injuries.

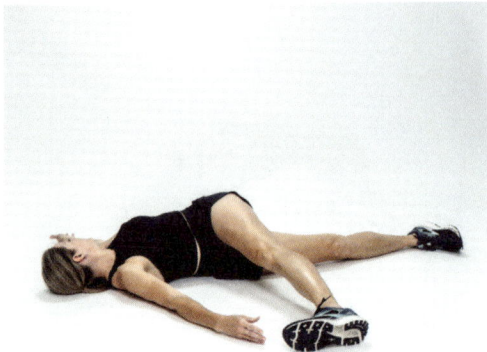

Lying Spinal Twist

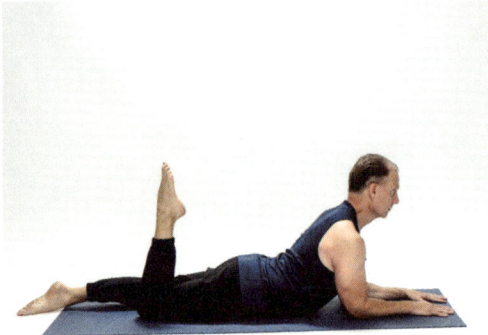

Single Leg Kick

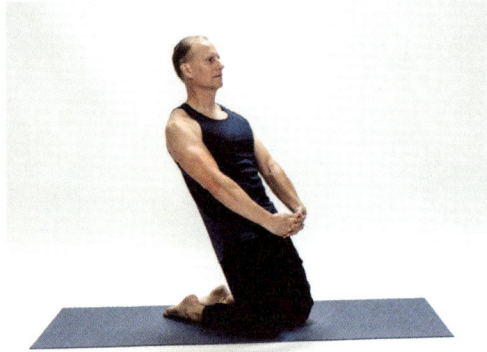

Camel Pulse

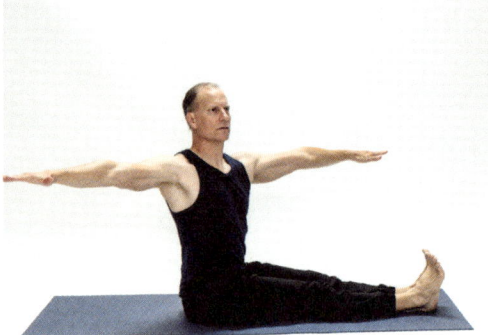

Spine Twist

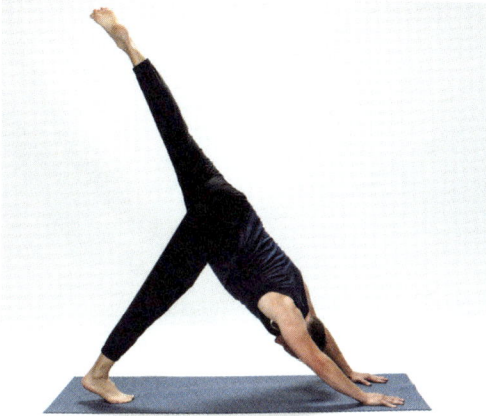

Down Dog Leg Lifts

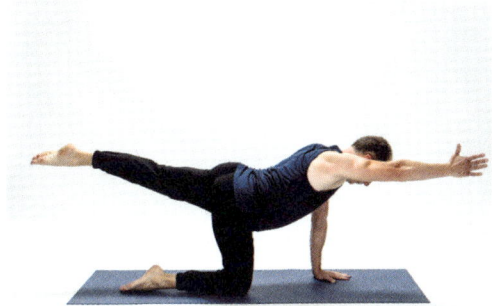

Birddog

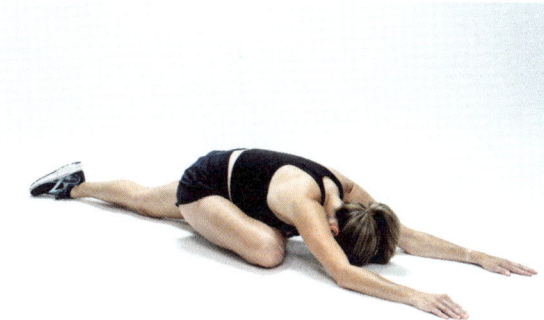

Pigeon

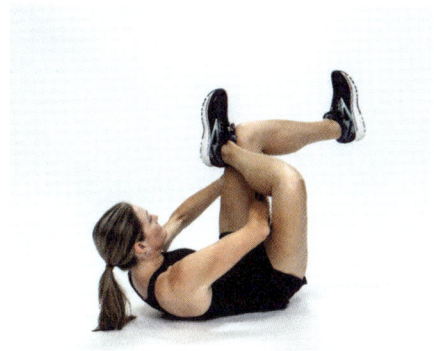

Figure Four

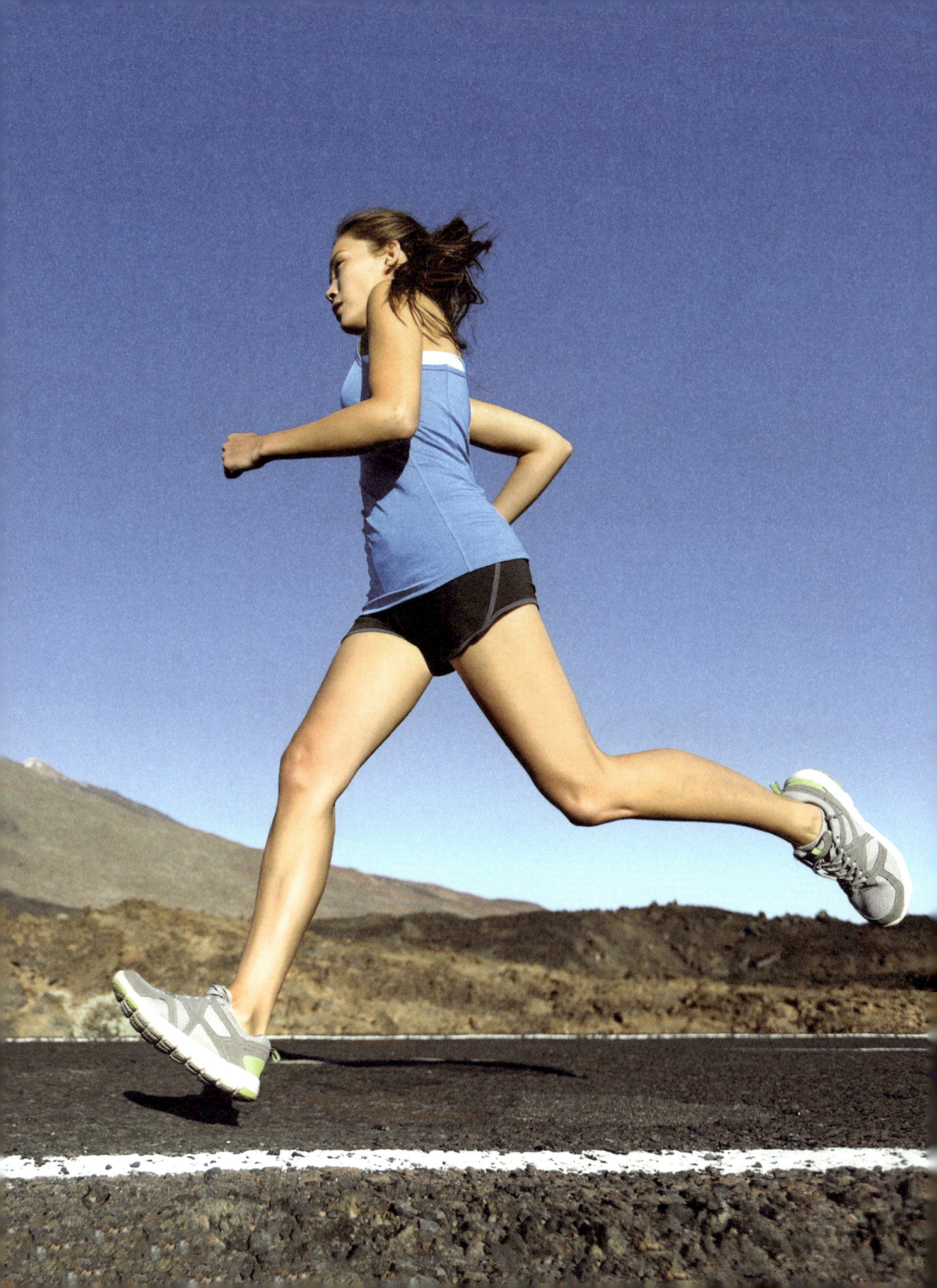

Resources

Want to continue your Pilates studies and keep that body moving like a well-oiled machine? You've come to the right place! Below, you'll find some of my favorite books to fuel and inspire your Pilates journey. No, there's no fancy diploma as you walk across the stage at the end but what you will earn is better movement, stronger muscles, smoother strides, and a whole lot more running power.

Bring your Pilates practice with you everywhere—on the mat, on the road, and into every run. Whether you're chasing a new PR or just running for the joy of it, Pilates is the secret sauce to reaching your goals and feeling amazing while you're at it.

Oh, and I've also included a few running-focused books that fired up my journey and might just do the same for you. I'd read them late at night and have trouble sleeping because I wanted to head outside and run, run, run. So, let's keep learning, keep moving, and keep having a blast doing it!

Isacowitz, Rael (2019). Pilates Anatomy. Human Kinetics

Karnazes, Dean (2006). *Ultramarathon Man: Confessions of an All-Night Runner.* TarcherPerigee

Karnazes, Dean (2022). *A Runner's High: My Life in Motion.* HarperOne

Lyon Jr, Daniel (2005). *The Complete Book of Pilates for Men: The Lifetime Plan for Strength, Power & Peak Performance.* Regan Books

McDougall, Christopher (2011). *Born to Run: A Hidden Tribe, Superathletes, and the Greatest Race the World Has Never Seen.* Vintage

Menezes, Alan (2004). *The Complete Guide to Joseph H. Pilates' Techniques of Physical Conditioning: With Special Help for Back Pain and Sports Training.* Hunter House

Vigue, Sean (2015). *Power Yoga for Athletes: More than 100 Poses and Flows to Improve Performance in Any Sport.* Fair Winds Press

Vigue, Sean (2021). Pilates for Athletes: *More than 200 Exercises and Flows to Improve Performance in Any Sport.* Hatherleigh Press

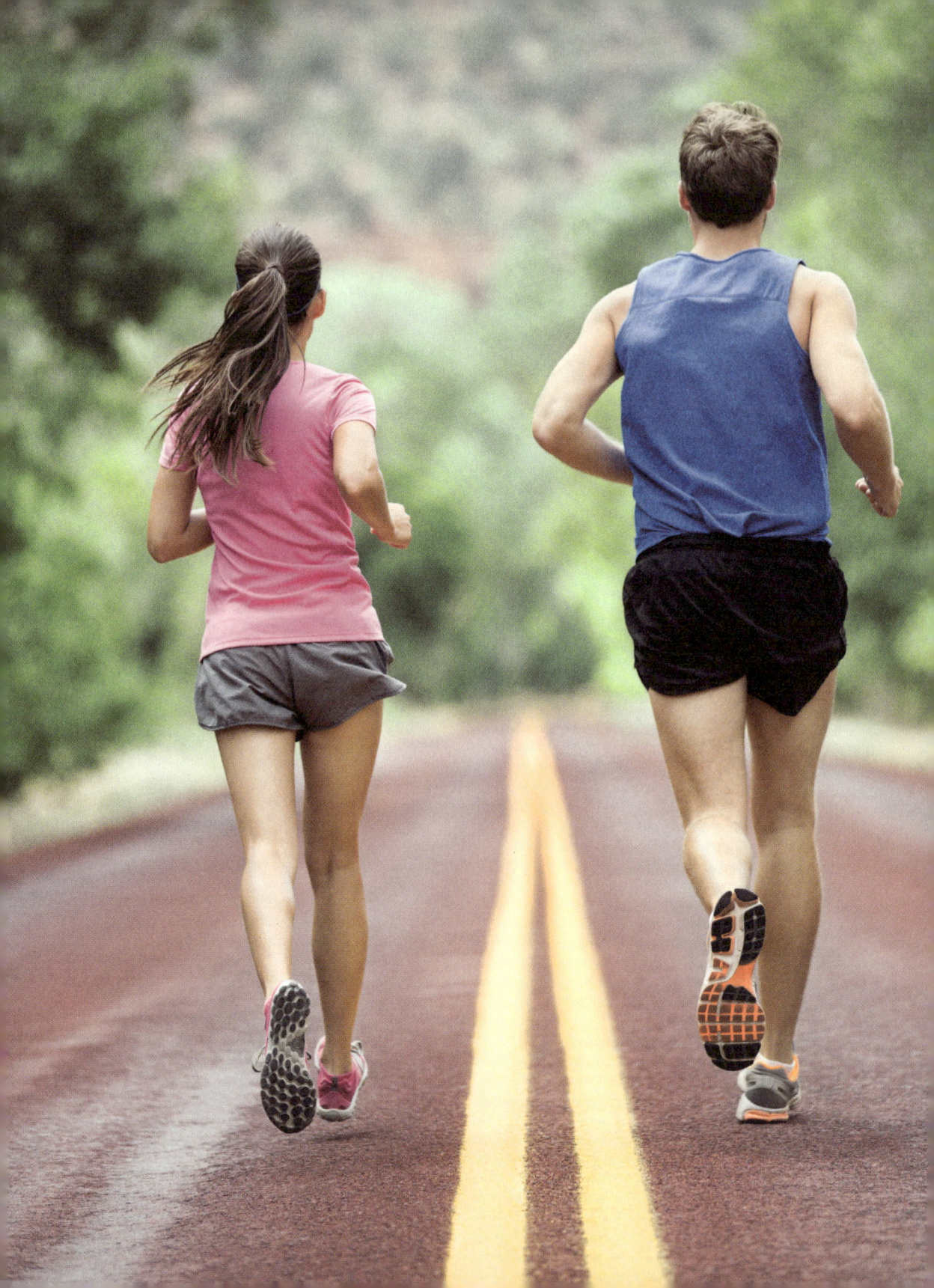

Going Further With Pilates

Once you've practiced and sufficiently mastered the exercises and flows in this book, I highly recommend expanding your Pilates universe! There's a whole world out there beyond the mat—Pilates styles that use equipment, machines, and odd-looking apparatuses that take your training to a whole new level.

Here are the top styles to explore next!

REFORMER PILATES

Now we're taking things up a notch with the Reformer—a sleek, spring-loaded machine that turns your body into a moving, stretching, strengthening masterpiece! Think resistance training meets graceful movement. This powerful machine provides adjustable tension, incredible range of motion, and a serious full body burn. It's like mat Pilates with turbo boosters (and jet pack) strapped to your abs. Smooth, strong, and studio-fancy.

CLASSICAL PILATES (No Equipment)

There's no school like the old school! Classical Pilates sticks to Joseph Pilates' original blueprint—34 exercises meant to be performed in a specific order, focusing on flowing movements, precision, breath, and control—each building on the last to work the entire body efficiently. You're flowing through exercises in a set sequence, practicing precision like a movement ninja. It's not flashy—it's pure, intentional, and powerful. Respect the roots, master the flow, and feel the fire in your core with every move. You can find more on this style in my previous book, *Pilates for Athletes*.

TOWER PILATES

This one's for the vertical thinkers! Tower Pilates uses a wall-mounted or Cadillac-style frame with push-through bars, springs, and loops to challenge your control from every angle. It's part strength training, part stretch therapy, and 100% mind-body magic. Hanging, pushing, pulsing; this style gives your core the royal treatment while pulling and lengthening muscles like a pro.

CHAIR PILATES WITH THE WUNDA CHAIR

Don't let the size fool you: the Wunda Chair packs a serious punch! It's basically a box with a spring-loaded pedal that demands balance, strength, and coordination all at once. Think squats, planks, presses, and splits all on one compact beast. The chair challenges your power-house with minimal surface area, meaning your stabilizers are forced to work overtime. You will sweat. You will shake. You will love it. You will quote Star Wars.

BARREL PILATES

This one is all about the stretch, the sculpt, and that sweet spinal alignment. Barrel Pilates uses rounded wooden or padded arc shapes to support your back, open your chest, and deepen your range of motion. It's super for doing backbends, core lifts, and leg stretches with flair. The Barrel helps you open up and find tremendous length like never before—think flexibility meeting fierce control.

PILATES FUSION

Time to mix it up with this style seen in a lot of gyms and health clubs to draw in new members. Pilates Fusion tosses tradition out the window (gently) and brings in a plethora of props to amplify the burn. Resistance bands for strength, Pilates rings for inner thighs of steel (and torture, so I've been told), stability balls for that delicious instability, and even light weights to amplify classical exercises and fire up your muscles. Fusion is wild—creative, dynamic, and always unpredictable. Your core will sing the Puccini high notes.

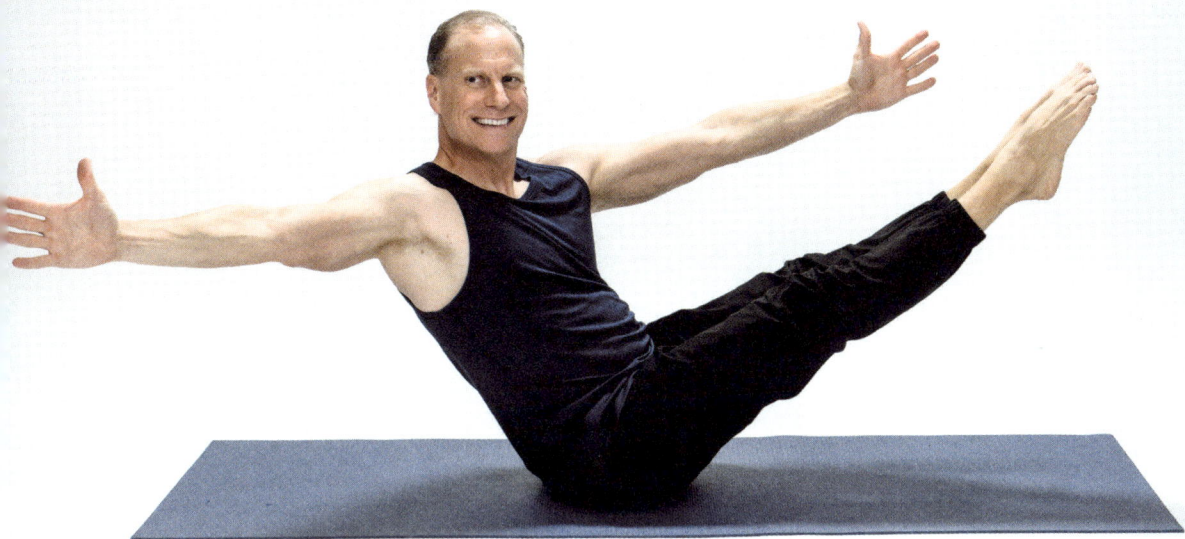

About the Author

Sean Vigue is an international fitness instructor and bestselling author known for making yoga, Pilates, and bodyweight training accessible to all. With a unique background in opera and musical theater, he brings unmatched energy, precision, and creativity to every workout. His bestselling books, including *Pilates for Athletes* and *Power Yoga for Athletes*, have helped thousands of readers build strength, flexibility, and endurance. Featured in countless publications including *The Washington Post, Fox News, Yoga Digest, Pilates Style* and *The Huffington Post*, Sean's expertise has reached millions through his books, YouTube channel, live classes and online classes. Whether you're a weekend warrior or elite athlete, Sean's guidance will challenge and inspire you every step of the way. He divides his time between Tennessee and Wisconsin with his wife, Jillian (the model in this book), son Dane and new puppy, Zuzu.

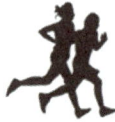

HEY RUNNER!

Ready to move better and feel stronger?

Scan the QR code to visit my site for exclusive *Pilates for Runners* workouts, bonus videos and details on joining Sean Vigue Fitness+.

Let's get to work!

seanviguefitness.com/pilates-for-runners

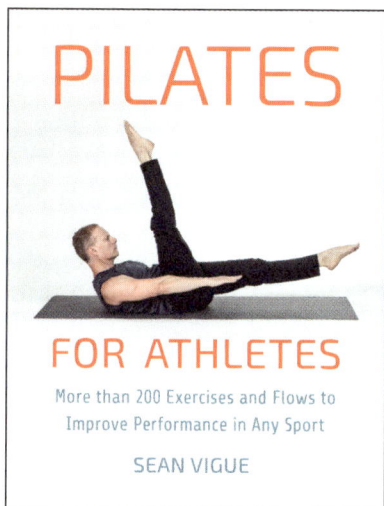

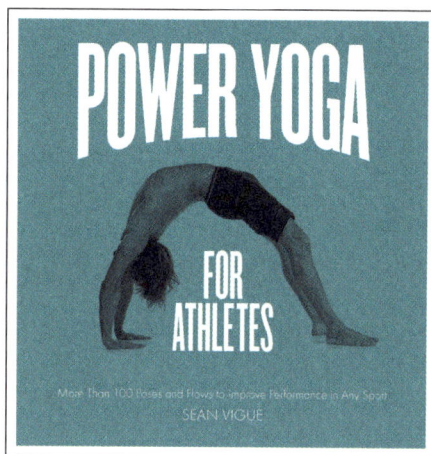

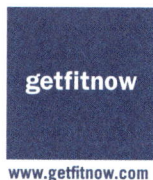

Index

YOUR TRAINING JOURNAL

YOUR TRAINING JOURNAL

YOUR TRAINING JOURNAL